THE ROAD
TO REFORM

THE ROAD TO REFORM

The Future of Health Care in America

ELI GINZBERG

with Miriam Ostow

THE FREE PRESS
A Division of Macmillan, Inc.
NEW YORK

Maxwell Macmillan Canada
TORONTO

Maxwell Macmillan International
NEW YORK   OXFORD   SINGAPORE   SYDNEY

The Free Press
A Division of Macmillan, Inc.
866 Third Avenue, New York, N.Y. 10022

Maxwell Macmillan Canada, Inc.
1200 Eglinton Avenue East
Suite 200
Don Mills, Ontario M3C 3N1

Macmillan, Inc. is part of the Maxwell Communication Group of Companies.

Printed in the United States of America

printing number

1 2 3 4 5 6 7 8 9 10

Library of Congress Cataloging-in-Publication Data

Ginzberg, Eli, 1911–
    The road to reform : the future of health care in America / Eli
Ginzberg with Miriam Ostow.
        p.   cm.
    Includes bibliographical references and index.
    ISBN 0–02-911715-1 : $22.95
    1. Health care reform—United States.   2. Medical policy—United
States.   I. Ostow, Miriam.   II. Title.
    RA395.A3G52   1994
    362.1′0973—dc20   93–48359
                                                                              CIP

For

ROBERT H. EBERT

Contents

1

Why This Book?

President Bill Clinton's speech on health reform to the joint session of the Congress in September 1993 was an unprecedented departure. No other chief executive had ever addressed the Congress on the subject of health reform. The Health Security Plan he proposed was, however, anything but new. The issue of national health insurance first surfaced at the presidential level in the 1912 election campaign, when Theodore Roosevelt, running a three-cornered race for the White House against William Howard Taft and Woodrow Wilson, supported it. From one perspective, Roosevelt's advocacy of national health insurance was farsighted, coming eight decades before Clinton put the matter directly before Congress with a strong recommendation for prompt action. In the annals of social legislation, however, it is worth observing that Chancellor Bismarck had taken the initial steps to establish national health insurance in Germany in 1883, almost thirty years before Theodore Roosevelt incorporated it in his platform.

A number of other stops along the way between 1912 and 1994 in the legislative journey of national health

insurance or universal coverage for medical care in the
United States warrant at least brief notice. The first and
most important was the New Deal. Although Franklin
Delano Roosevelt considered writing national health insurance into the Social Security legislation of 1935, he
decided that it was the better part of wisdom not to,
faced as he was with the determined opposition of the
American Medical Association (AMA), the antagonism of
the business community, and the absence of any large
bloc of supporters among the public at large. FDR con-
cluded that the introduction of national health insurance
coverage could jeopardize the passage of the rest of his
reforms, a risk he decided not to take.

The half-century since World War II has seen periodic
approaches by various presidents to health care reform,
particularly national health insurance, but until President
Clinton's historic address, the issue was never central to
the legislative agendas of the successive administrations
or able to engage and hold the attention of the electorate.
For example, shortly after the end of World War II, President Harry Truman sent a message to Congress urging
the enactment of national health insurance. And in the
late 1940s several liberal Democratic members of the
House and Senate sought to advance the legislation but
failed to elicit any broad-based support, even from the
rank and file of American workers.

Starting in 1929 and growing slowly during the
depressed 1930s, regional Blue Cross plans offered Americans an opportunity for protection against the prospective high costs of hospitalization by enrolling in a
prepayment plan that was usually open to everyone at a
uniform community-based premium. This private, nonprofit health insurance system underwent rapid growth

during World War II when the federal government agreed that unions could bargain for health care benefits without violating the prevailing wage freeze. Its expansion was stimulated by the federal tax code; employer premium payments for health insurance benefits were treated as a nontaxable business expense, and the value of the benefits was exempted from the income tax liability of the recipient.

The chief reason that the Truman proposal for national health insurance failed to be enacted was the growing enthusiasm of both labor and employers for private health insurance that held the promise of providing coverage for catastrophic medical expenditures without requiring the much enlarged engagement of the federal government to accomplish this desirable and desired national goal.

The growth of nongovernmental health insurance was accelerated in the 1950s by the aggressive efforts of commercial health insurance companies, which offered employers a better deal by quoting a premium rate based on the employer's individual experience, not a community rate that was the practice of the Blue Cross plans. An employer with a relatively young work force, in an industry with a low frequency of accident and illness, could usually purchase health care benefits for employees more cheaply from the commercial companies than from the Blue Cross plans. Eventually most Blue Cross plans were forced by competitive pressures to offer employers experience-rated premiums also, thus setting the stage for the increasing difficulties that the elderly, the chronically ill, and others at high risk would encounter in obtaining coverage at a price that they could afford.

By the late 1950s, another serious shortcoming of private health insurance emerged. The system was founded on employment; health insurance was a fringe benefit added to workers' wages. This meant that those who stopped working because of age or disability were no longer covered, just at the point in life when they had an increasing need for health care.

When John F. Kennedy ran for the presidency in 1960, one plank in his platform was the early enactment of Medicare, a tax-based insurance system to provide health care coverage to the elderly, defined as those over age sixty-five. Confronted by the unyielding resistance of the AMA to a federally funded health insurance system and the ideological antagonism of fiscal conservatives in the Democratic party, Kennedy was unable to persuade Congress to act on his proposal. After his resounding victory over Senator Barry Goldwater in 1964, Lyndon Baines Johnson, however, succeeded in getting Medicare passed and, what is more, Medicaid, a joint federal-state program to ensure access to health care for selected categories of the poor, particularly women and children on welfare. The prevailing view among the liberal political leadership was that the passage of Medicare and Medicaid represented the first phase in the implementation of national health insurance; a bill to cover health care services for all women and children would come next, and not long thereafter all adult men would be covered, completing the circle of universal coverage for the American people.

Despite the scale and scope of the Great Society programs, President Johnson gave no serious consideration to the enactment of national health insurance. The public recognized the urgent need to ensure continuing coverage for persons who were no longer in the labor force, but they found no reason to discard private health insurance for the employed population and their dependents. Accordingly, legislation to provide health insurance for women and children was never enacted.

The early to mid-1970s saw a renewed interest in health reform and national health insurance by three successive presidents: Nixon, Ford, and Carter. Interest yes, but action no. Both the White House and the Congress had come to appreciate within a few years of the implementation of Medicare and Medicaid (in 1966) that the cost projections for both programs had been seriously understated. With the passage of time, it also became clear that private health insurance plus Medicare plus Medicaid still left substantial numbers of persons without any form of coverage for shorter or longer periods of time.

Had it not been for the distraction of Watergate and the inflexibility of the southern Democrats, the United States might have passed in the early 1970s a system of universal coverage consisting of expanded employer coverage, supplemented by government-financed coverage for those not insured through employment—a compromise between the alternative proposals of President Nixon and Senator Ted Kennedy. By the time that President Ford first recommended the enactment of national health insurance, the federal budget and inflation added powerful new disincentives that persuaded him not to resubmit his recommendation.

Like his Democratic predecessors, Jimmy Carter included a plank in his 1976 presidential campaign platform favoring national health insurance, but once again money came between social commitment and legislative realities. Shortly after he took office, his advisers persuaded him that there was no possible way for him to obtain the necessary congressional support. The tens of billions of additional dollars required to turn national health insurance from a goal into an operative program could not be drawn from the American taxpayer. In that year, 1977, federal spending for health care amounted to about $47 billion, or 13.2 percent of total federal expenditures. (Let us put these figures into perspective: in 1993, total federal outlays for health care amounted to $286 billion, or 19.7 percent of total budgetary outlays.)

For the better part of two decades, that is from the early 1970s until the 1990s, major health reform all but disappeared from the presidential and national agendas, preoccupied as the country was with inflation, the cold war, and economic expansion. Although both Presidents Reagan and Bush had to respond to a great number of specific challenges growing out of the need of the federal government to slow its steeply rising expenditures for Medicare and Medicaid, the twelve years of Republican leadership in Washington were marked by a studied avoidance of any large-scale national health reform.

Why then did Bill Clinton, first as candidate and then as White House incumbent, single out health reform as a priority goal of his administration? There was nothing in the past or more recent history of the United States to suggest that a president who was elected with only 43 percent of the popular vote would be able to accomplish what none of his predecessors—including FDR, Johnson, Nixon, and Reagan, who won with overwhelming popular support—had been willing to tackle. How is 1994 different from 1981, 1973, 1965, or 1935?

The answer is both simple and complicated. The simple version can point to the growing numbers of individuals who have fallen between the cracks in the extant systems of payment for health care—private insurance and governmentally financed programs. At any time, about 37 million Americans are without health care coverage, and the figure has been rising slowly but steadily over the past decade. However, our history and political experience offer little reason to believe that the majority of the American people who today have good private or public coverage would advocate or support a radical transformation of the nation's health care system to ensure that the small minority—14 percent of their fellow citizens—should be similarly covered. True, they have indicated on opinion surveys their approval of a national initiative to provide universal coverage and even a willingness to pay somewhat more taxes in order to accomplish this goal. However, they have given no indication that their concern for the uninsured would make them strong supporters of fundamental health care reforms. Why, then, has President Clinton designated health reform as a key commitment of his administration? *Why 1994?*

During his presidential campaign, during the interval that he was president-elect, and during the early months of his administration, as he, Hillary Rodham Clinton, and his staff were refining the details of his reform proposals, the President provided insights as to why early and comprehensive reforms were needed. In his speech to the Congress in September 1993, the President reviewed the entire terrain, emphasizing the reasons that major health reform could no longer be delayed.

He stated boldly that our health care system was badly broken, that it needed fixing, and that we had wasted decades in false starts to reform it. He identified the worst failings of the system:

- Millions of Americans are at risk of losing their private health insurance coverage.
- The cost of financing the system is twice the rate of growth of the gross domestic product (GDP).
- The United States spends about one-third more than other nations that rank *below* it on the spending curve.
- The U.S. system wastes substantial amounts of money it can no longer afford.

To address these faults, the President identified six goals of reform: security, simplicity, savings, choice, quality and responsibility.

With respect to security, the President urged the Congress to act promptly to adopt a system of universal coverage that would ensure every American lifetime entitlement to essential health care services. Guaranteed coverage would include access to preventive care, retention of the Medicare program for the elderly, and the phasing in of long-term care and home care for the disabled and the elderly.

On the issue of simplicity, the President emphasized the need to make the current system more user friendly for patients, physicians and other providers, and insurers. A principal mechanism would be the introduction of a universal form that would provide an account of the services that the patient received and would also serve as his or her basic bill.

The President was unequivocal in his insistence on significant savings. He found no justification for the United States to spend 14 percent or more of GDP for health care when no other nation exceeds 9 percent. In exploring the options for achieving the required savings, the President indicated that he favored intensified competition over fee controls. If intensified competition failed to rein in price increases, the federal government would limit the rate of premium increases to ensure that total spending was constrained. The President called for the elimination of the historic practice of cross-subsidization, the custom of hospitals to balance their outlays and their revenues by "overcharging" some customers (those with good private health insurance) by some 20 to 30 percent to compensate for the shortfalls that accrue as a result of the failure of other payers, primarily government, to reimburse them fully for the patient care that they provide. Shortfalls resulting from bad debts and charity care are also loaded on to the bills of the well insured. It is obvious that cross-subsidization perversely penalizes employers that provide workers with health care benefits. Clinton also stressed vigorously the need to rid the current system of waste generated by excessive paperwork, malpractice insurance and litigation, and fraud and abuse amounting to perhaps $200 billion annually.

With respect to his remaining three goals of choice, quality, and responsibility, the President argued that under our health care system, individuals are deprived of choice because many corporations offer their employees only one health care plan. Physicians as well as patients could benefit from wider choices and should have the option of joining alternative plans.

In the determination of quality, the President noted the dearth of consumer information on the relative efficiency and efficacy of alternative procedures; fee scales, for example, are not a reliable guide to quality of care. Under the reformed system, the American public would have the ability to rate providers. The President also promised that his search for efficiency and economy would not result in the underfunding of biomedical research and development, which continue to offer the best prospect for more effective responses to the major health threats.

The final goal of shared responsibility was conveyed by an appeal to the American people. Everyone must contribute to the financing of the system; the nation must alter its behavior on a series of fronts—smoking, teenage sex, AIDS, violence, and other social and clinical pathologies; and every individual must accept personal responsibility for his or her health.

In his conclusion the President returned to the financing of his plan and its potential costs to the public. He reassured small businesses that they would be assisted by a phase-in period and by special government subsidies to cover their employees; he reassured the self-employed that they would have a 100 percent tax deduction to help them cover their insurance premiums; and he reassured all citizens that no new taxes would be levied other than on cigarettes.

The President has declared that the nation dare not continue in the evasive and avoidance mode that it has followed since the early 1970s, when major health reform last occupied a serious place on the domestic agenda. Total health care spending is out of control; federal and state budgets are increasingly strained by ever larger appropriations for health; American employers are handicapped in competing in the world markets because of their galloping health care benefit costs; and, to add insult to injury, 37 million Americans are uninsured, and millions more fear that they will be deprived of coverage at some time in the future. Overall the system is characterized by complexity, waste, fraud, and abuse, which impede the delivery of quality care. In the President's view, the nation must weigh the costs of staying on its present course versus the costs of change, and he urged the American people to write a new chapter in the American health care story.

This brings us to the second question in the chapter's title: *Why this book?* Quite simply, President Clinton has thrown down the gauntlet and placed major health reform at the top of the nation's agenda (and at the heart of his political career). No matter what the response of the American people and the Congress will be—enactment, modification, rejection, or any combination thereof—health reform will remain a focus of social policy for the foreseeable future. The reasons will become evident in the concluding chapter. This being the case, it is necessary that all interested and concerned Americans become well informed about the complex set of forces that drive the current health care system, that they understand how health care policy has been defined in the past by the interactions among the major parties of interest, and that they assess intelligently the responses and reactions of the key parties to the Clinton proposals.

This book was written specifically to inform the concerned public, not a handful of experts, about the major transformations that the U.S. health care system has undergone in the four decades since 1950 as it expanded from 4.5 percent of GDP to over 14 percent in 1993. Unless the public gains a deeper insight into the forces that have propelled the U.S. health care system to the point where it will pierce the trillion-dollar level by the end of 1994, providing employment for 10 million workers ranging from neurosurgeons to hospital housekeeping staff, it will be poorly positioned to communicate to the Congress its primary goals for reform and its preferences among competing mechanisms. When confronted by a major challenge—and no sensible person would question that reform of the health care system is a national challenge—a democratic people does not have the option of ceding the solution to elected or appointed officials. Access to health care is too critical to leave the outcome to the major interest groups and the members of Congress.

One way for the concerned American public to participate intelligently in the contentious process of reaching a consensus on the reforms that must be introduced is to examine critically the actions of the major parties in response to past efforts to alter the existing health care system. The answers that we seek may not be found in the earlier actions of Congress to reform the system and the consequences of their efforts. Obviously, had the earlier answers been more apposite and effective, we would not now be facing what the President has defined as a broken system. Nevertheless, ignorance and misinformation about how the United States has responded to past challenges will deprive us of a major source of guidance in responding today. By interpreting what went before, this book hopes to contribute to the sophistication of concerned citizen-voters about the cacophony of arguments and contentions to which they will be exposed during the debate over the health care system.

Deficits and shortcomings in the financing and delivery of health care are, however, only part of the story. There are also impressive accomplishments of the health care system that have propelled the United States into a position of leadership in terms of the quantity and quality of health care services available to the majority of its population that enjoys good insurance coverage. The United States has in place the most advanced biomedical research enterprise in the world, and its pharmaceutical industry is unparalleled. Its acute care hospitals are better equipped and staffed than those of any other nation. Clearly there is much about the U.S. health care sector that commands the respect and admiration of those at home and abroad and should be preserved and strengthened.

The principal thrust of the book is to provide nonspecialist readers with a sufficiently detailed and documented account of how a relatively minor sector of the American economy, amounting prior to World War II to around 4 percent of the GDP, was radically expanded and elaborated in the postwar decades so that it currently accounts for one-seventh of the nation's output, on the way to one-fifth by, probably, the end of this decade. Underlying this spectacular growth of the health care sector are a series of important systemic developments; we will identify these, trace their evolution, and assess their impact.

First was the decision of the federal government shortly after the end of World War II to initiate a broad-based program for the support of biomedical research, whose productive potential was an unanticipated inference that emerged from the nation's wartime experience. An ample flow of resources, personnel, and capital was directed to research in the expectation of high and continuing returns in the form of new knowledge and new techniques that would provide the underlying dynamism for the continuing elaboration and transformation of our health care system.

Rapid expansion of the physician supply was a second transformational development. Nonprofit universities and state governments had historically been responsible for educating and training young people to enter the medical profession; the numbers admitted and the educational standards were largely under the control of the medical profession. In the post–World War II decades, there was growing pressure from many different constituencies to expand the nation's medical school capacity in order to correct the widely perceived shortage of physicians. These pressures led to major construction and financing programs, first by the states and later by the federal government. Because of the considerable lag time between the approval of a new medical school and the production of its first graduating class, Congress found a more immediate mechanism to respond to the mounting demand for more physicians: modification of the U.S. immigration statutes to permit the admission of physicians (foreign nationals) who had been trained abroad. Few people are aware that one of every four physicians now in active practice in the United States obtained his or her medical degree in another country.

A third revolutionizing trend, also dating from the post–World War II years, was the substantial investment in the construction, modernization, and upgrading of teaching and community hospitals, which have become the centers for sophisticated medical treatment. Both federal and state governments made significant amounts of public dollars available to supplement and augment the sizable sums that hospital trustees could raise to enlarge and improve the nation's hospital plant.

The restructuring of health care financing was still

another catalyzing development. At the end of World War II, most Americans paid for their health care out of pocket. Physicians took care of the poor by treating them at a nominal fee or without charge. Most hospitals provided a substantial amount of inpatient care to individuals in marginal economic circumstances free of charge or at reduced rates. Public hospitals, most of them run by the county or the state, served primarily the urban or rural poor. Nevertheless, a significant proportion of the low-income population had little or no access to the health care system.

With hospital care becoming more critical to modern medical practice and with hospital costs rising as a consequence of new and improved technology and more highly skilled personnel, the costs of hospitalization became an increasing burden for patients who paid out of pocket for their care. World War II saw the rapid expansion of private health insurance for hospital care, a fringe benefit that more and more employers offered in lieu of wage increases.

Under the combined stimuli of expanding research and development, the growing physician supply, the enlargement and upgrading of the nation's hospital plant, and the growing source of new funding from private health insurance, the U.S. health care system underwent a substantial reorientation. The volume and sophistication of the services it provided the American people by the 1990s would have been unimaginable in the 1930s.

Many among the designers of the Great Society reforms saw Medicare and Medicaid as major building blocks positioning the nation on its way to national health insurance. Although that scenario did not play out, there was a substantial increase in the demand for hospital, physician, and other health services, fueled by the new federal and state dollars that turned large numbers of charity patients into cash-paying consumers. In fact, the new sources of funding soon became a matter of increasing concern to the federal government, state governments, employers, and eventually households— that is, all of the principal payers. For the better part of the 1970s and the 1980s, government and employers explored a variety of initiatives aimed at the singular goal of moderating their annual outlays for health care expenditures, which were increasing at a rate that seriously compromised their ability to meet other priority commitments. These efforts were to no avail: The nation's spending for health care continued to rise at a rate two to three times that of the economy at large.

The unarrested explosion of health care expenditures was paralleled by another development: Increasing numbers of Americans—currently 37 million, or 15 percent of the population—lack insurance coverage, and many more millions will find themselves in the same predicament in the next year or two. Clearly, there is something fundamentally wrong with the U.S. health care system if it spends considerably more per capita and in total than any other advanced nation yet fails to provide basic coverage for its entire citizenry, a commitment that all of the other advanced nations have long since made and delivered on.

The singularity of the U.S. health care system, particularly its shortcomings, has not been lost on the American public. Debate about the desirability and the direction of health care reform in this country can no longer be conducted without reference to what is happening in other industrialized societies—specifically our northern neighbor, Canada, with its single payer-system, and Germany, much farther away, which appears to share some structural characteristics with our decentralized, employment-based insurance system. However, looking for useful lessons in the experience of foreign lands must not overlook the incontestable fact that every nation's health care system is inextricably linked to its unique history, institutions, societal characteristics, and politics. Comparative assessments that do not take account of these powerful, if unquantifiable, factors are of questionable validity. And direct borrowing is exceedingly difficult, if not impossible. Consider the differences that are manifest when the United States looks closely at the Canadian experience: We have more than ten times Canada's population; we have much greater racial and ethnic diversity; we are skeptical, if not suspicious, of government as an engine of reform, while the Canadians have much greater confidence in the potential of government. U.S. physicians have long enjoyed much higher incomes than their Canadian colleagues; Canada has only a modest biomedical research enterprise; its hospitals are, on average, less technologically advanced. Moreover, the entire population of Canada could be absorbed by the state of California with room to spare. And these are just a few of the differences. It simply does not make a great deal of sense to emulate Canada's system.

Few Americans fully appreciate not only how different our health care system is from those of other advanced nations but, even more important, the extent to which our system has evolved along distinctive lines, quite unlike other major sectors of the economy and the society. Consider first the economy. Ours is overwhelmingly market oriented; the public relies on profit-seeking enterprises to provide it with the goods and services that it wants, and at a competitive price. The public's consumption is limited by the amount of income that it is able and willing to direct to the goods offered in comparison with other goods that it also desires.

In addition to its overwhelming reliance on the competitive market, the American public obtains a limited number of goods and services directly through the instrumentality of government. It pays taxes and expects from government a range of critical services ranging from defense to education, highway maintenance, police, and social services for the indigent. Our health care system—which, it must be recalled, accounts for one-seventh of the total national economy—fits neither model. It is not specifically dependent on the competitive market, nor is it a direct tax-based public service enterprise. Rather, it is a uniquely pluralistic system.

To appreciate the character of this pluralistic system, consider the following: Is there another category of consumption in which the individual obtains routine services via prepayment (insurance) and the (insured) purchaser is freed of concern about the amount or quality of the goods and services that he or she chooses to consume?

Admittedly, many of the producers or providers of the goods and services that the public needs and wants operate in accordance with the design of the competitive market, seeking to produce at the lowest possible combination of cost and quality sufficient to attract the business of the purchasers. That, however, does not apply to one of the largest subsectors of the health care industry, hospitals. Economy in the utilization of resources does not determine the quality, characteristics or volume of the services they produce.

When it comes to capital expenditures for expansion or modernization, most large teaching and university hospitals are able to borrow the bulk of the funds they need from the bond market, where their bonds enjoy special tax treatment. Although hospitals in the same geographic area undeniably compete, competition is based for the most part not on price, or even on price and quality combined, but primarily on professional reputation, which translates into the ability to attract to their staff prominent, prestigious physicians and surgeons. To do so, they seek constantly to acquire the most advanced equipment and services, with the result that most market areas are characterized by a large amount of expensive, underutilized technology.

Further, by state statute and regulation, only licensed physicians are permitted to provide medical care to the public. At the same time, physicians have discretion over the location where they choose to live and practice, and as a consequence large numbers of low-income urban and rural residents have been seriously underserved. The competitive market has failed to distribute the physician supply according to need, and government, both federal and state, has not intervened effectively to correct the perverseness of the market.

There is no analogue in the American economy for the mechanisms that govern the production and distribution of health care services to the American people. The mechanisms of private health insurance, public health insurance (Medicare and Medicaid), and self-pay represent a unique payment constellation. Similarly unique is the dependence of the health care system on the operations and interactions of a vast institutional infrastructure established and managed variously by the three sectors: nonprofit, profit, and government.

The chapters that follow analyze the major forces that have determined the evolution of this distinctive health care delivery system. Such an understanding is an essential point of departure in seeking reforms that can no longer be delayed.

2

What's Right About the Health Care System?

The press has been increasingly preoccupied with accounts of all that is wrong, often seriously wrong, with the U.S. health care system. Without denying the legitimacy of the many complaints and criticisms, it is important to remember that much is also right with our health care delivery system. The merits and strengths of the system need to be recognized, if only to ensure that in some headlong effort at reform, we do not undermine characteristics and values that should be preserved and reinforced.

Americans who are preparing for a stint overseas or a trip abroad invariably face the question of how and where to seek medical care in case of serious illness or injury. The tentative answers depend on the continents and countries that are on the itinerary and, of course, the nature of the disease or disability that occurs. In the early postwar decades, more often than not the choice was to return, whenever possible, to the United States for definitive treatment. Even now, in the 1990s, a prompt flight to the United States remains for most Americans, physicians and nonphysicians alike, the preferred avenue.

This decision might seem to reflect an overvaluation of the quality of medical treatment in the United States or a hypercritical view of the quality of care available in other advanced nations, but the judgment is not seriously awry. One conclusion is unequivocal: In a serious emergency, admission to a hospital selected at random in the United Kingdom, France, Germany, or Italy is far less advisable than admission to a major teaching hospital in the United States.

The significant advantage that the United States has over other advanced countries is the much higher probability that a teaching hospital of reasonable size will be well staffed by an array of specialists and subspecialists, with appropriate support personnel and advanced technology at their disposal. The 1,200 teaching hospitals in the United States, and particularly the 320 members of the Council of Teaching Hospitals, are in a position to provide all patients whom they admit medical care that is probably superior in quality to that available anywhere else in the world. This was not always the case, but it has become increasingly so during the past quarter century in which there has been a marked upgrading of the capability of acute care hospitals in medium-sized and even smaller communities throughout the United States, undergirded by a massive expansion in the number of well-trained physicians.

It is worth noting that the continental United States, a land mass of more than 3 million square miles, is larger in area than all four principal Western European countries (Great Britain, France, Germany, and Spain) combined and that its population of 260 million exceeds their combined total. One of the striking achievements of the United States during the past decades has been the establishment of a uniformly high standard of physician care and acute hospital care that is available to most, if not all, Americans.

Another major source of strength of the U.S. health care system has been the leadership that the federal government assumed at the end of World War II in becoming the principal funder of basic biomedical research. It has carried out this role primarily in direct association with the nation's leading universities and medical schools and indirectly with the for-profit pharmaceutical and medical supply companies. The trend in research funding has been uninterruptedly in one direction, up, to a national level currently approaching $30 billion annually. The substantial advances in the biomedical knowledge base have been the foundation for steady progress in the clinical treatment of a wide variety of previously fatal or crippling diseases and have produced corresponding gains in the quality of life of the elderly (as well as of many younger persons) and in the average longevity of both men and women. Throughout the post-World War II decades, the biomedical research effort in the United States has far outpaced that of the rest of the industrial world, although recently Germany and Japan have begun to compete by substantially increasing their research outlays.

It is often contended that the emphasis in the health care community on high-tech medicine and the rapid development and diffusion of new modes of diagnosis and treatment is intrinsically flawed. The human life span appears to have an upper limit (it is rare for an individual to live past age one hundred), and, the argument goes, if one does not die of cancer or stroke, the likely alternative is heart disease or other organ failure.

Given the certainty of death and the possibility of only modest palliatives once chronic disease and organ failure develop, what is the rationale for the all but limitless effort that the United States directs to advancing the frontiers of medicine through research and the translation of the knowledge gained into new diagnostic and therapeutic techniques? Wouldn't investments in improving the everyday conditions of life—replacing substandard housing, upgrading public education, providing employment for all—have greater social utility? This challenge has been definitively answered by the American people, who have repeatedly affirmed through their government and their pocketbooks their commitment to the continuing advancement of medical knowledge that leads to improved medical treatment. Faced with the alternative of loss of productivity, pain, debilitation, and premature death, the public continues to vote for prolonging independence and functionality, surcease from pain, and delaying death.

Relatively little attention has been paid to the vast post–World War II expansion of the biomedical R&D enterprise in the United States, supported with federal funds and conducted through informal, highly productive relations with the leading academic health centers on the one hand and with private, profit-seeking pharmaceutical and medical equipment manufacturing companies on the other. Once Congress decided to direct most of the new federal appropriations to the support of external research, the leading academic health centers were quick to respond. Moreover, the pharmaceutical and medical supply companies, both the well-established large corporations and the many new venture capital and small firms, set themselves the task of translating the new research discoveries into useful products, which they sought to diffuse expeditiously to hospitals, physicians, and patients. With the advantage of hindsight, one is impressed with the comparative ease with which these critical linkages were forged among the government, academia, and the for-profit sector, relationships that have continued to operate, at least until recently, with relatively little friction.

A further accommodation that the U.S. system was able to make quite early—possibly too early—was the striking expansion of the graduate medical education system, which helped to train the large number of specialists and subspecialists that the sophisticated advances on the research and clinical fronts required. There is a growing consensus that the academic health centers overshot the mark and that today there are too many subspecialists and too few generalists, an issue that will be considered in the next chapter. For now, in assessing the strengths of the United States system, suffice it to say that the rapid elaboration of graduate medical education was the enabling factor without which U.S. medicine could not have reached the pinnacle of clinical excellence it now occupies.

A signal strength of the graduate medical education structure has been the substantial freedom of choice permitted the young physician-in-training in deciding which of the many fields of specialization or subspecialization to enter. True, there are limits to the choice since the number of residency slots is prescribed and the competition for preferred training opportunities intense. Nevertheless, compared with most other advanced countries, the opportunities for able students to chart their training programs and consequently their professional careers are considerably greater in the United States than elsewhere. Although this freedom has its costs, it also has the advantage of contributing to a better match between the individual's capacities and interests and his or her career objectives.

Notwithstanding the substantial changes in the intensity, sophistication, and breadth of health care services provided to the American people during the past several decades, the normative career mode for physicians has remained the same: independent practice, solo or as a member of a group. Apparently, most physicians and most patients believe that this traditional mode of practice—patients, provided they have good insurance coverage, are free to select a physician and physicians compete with one another to attract and retain patients—is preferable to employment by government or by a corporate enterprise. Patient option in the selection of physician(s) continues to be a valued attribute of the American health care system, one that is not available in many other countries. Most foreign health care systems differentiate between physicians who provide ambulatory care (generalists) and those with a hospital appointment (specialists), and patients are permitted to consult specialists only with the authorization of their regular physician.

A unique characteristic of the U.S. health care system has been the dominant role that voluntary hospitals have played in providing both inpatient and ambulatory care in many urban areas to indigent patients who are unable to pay the costs incurred and must be subsidized in whole or in part. This voluntary tradition dates back to the eighteenth century, which saw the beginnings of philanthropically supported community hospitals in Philadelphia and New York. It is worth noting that ever since 1771, when the Society of the New York Hospital received its original charter, voluntary contributions to hospital revenues have been frequently supplemented by legislative grants. Such commingling of funding streams has been a feature of hospital financing from colonial times to the present.

The continuing role of eleemosynary groups in the establishment and operation of community hospitals is distinctive to the United States. Many institutions were founded by religious or ethnic groups that considered it their responsibility to provide hospital care for their coreligionists and conationals, particularly those who could not afford to pay. The humanitarian motives of the various sectarian and ethnic charitable organizations were reinforced by the perceived need to provide training opportunities and admitting privileges for young physicians of specific national (non-Anglo-Saxon) and religious (non-Protestant) origins, who were generally discriminated against by mainstream institutions.

In the early part of the twentieth century, when hospitalization became an essential element in the provision of health care to the middle class, a major spur to the establishment of community hospitals was the antigovernmental political culture of American society. The growth of social welfare institutions, not least hospitals, was perceived to be a function of private philanthropy, not a public function. The record speaks for itself. Of the 3,940 nongovernmental acute care hospitals accredited by the Joint Commission on Accreditation of Healthcare Organizations, 3,191 (81 percent) are under voluntary auspices (the remaining 19 percent are for-profit); the voluntary sector's share of total bed capacity in these hospitals, 87 percent, is even more impressive.

Notwithstanding the major post-World War II shift following the passage of the Hospital Survey and Construction Act of 1946, popularly known as the Hill-Burton Act, which committed the federal government to large-scale financial assistance for the expansion of community hospitals, most of the needed capital funds continued to be raised by community leaders. The voluntary hospital system, for its part, underwent a series of major transformations, most of them unanticipated, others unnecessary, and some dysfunctional. The rapid escalation of hospital costs subsequent to the passage of Medicare and Medicaid made it increasingly difficult for voluntary hospitals to continue to provide significant amounts of charity care, that is, services to patients with no insurance or other means of paying their hospital bill. Further, as per diem costs of tertiary hospital care climbed to nearly $1,000 (1992), voluntary hospitals have seen no option but to institute tight management practices focused on budgets, expenditures, and surpluses. In short, voluntary hospitals have come to resemble the for-profit hospital sector, which expanded rapidly following the institution of Medicare and Medicaid. The historic philanthropic mission of voluntary hospitals has been seriously eroded.

These significant evolutionary changes have, nevertheless, served one important function: Voluntary hospitals have continued to offer an alternative to government monopoly over the ownership and management of acute care hospitals that is found in most other advanced countries. Aneurin Bevan, the Minister of Health of the United Kingdom, who designed the National Health Service in the late 1940s, observed at the time that it was the financial exhaustion of the British voluntary hospitals that added momentum and support for the national government to take over the restructuring of the British health care system.

In identifying the comparative strengths of the U.S. hospital system in the early 1990s, the following factors are important. First and foremost, the predominance of the voluntary sector continues. About two-thirds of all acute care beds are under voluntary control; the remainder is divided between government and the for-profit sector in a ratio of two to one. The voluntary sector, with important assistance from the government, has been able to provide the American public with a broad spectrum of acute care hospital services. Moreover, informed observers agree that the quality of care in most of the voluntary hospitals is superior to that available elsewhere in the industrialized world and is generally superior to the care provided in the public and for-profit hospitals in the United States that serve the remaining third of the population.

Unlike the academic health centers, whose major teaching hospital(s) are staffed primarily by medical school faculty, voluntary commmunity hospitals have been willing to open their facilities to all qualified physicians in the area rather than rely exclusively or primarily on a full-time hospital staff, which is the norm in Germany, the United Kingdom and many other countries. This practice has tended to improve the quality of care provided by community practitioners and has been reassuring to patients, who know that their personal physician will be able to follow their progress and to counsel them during a hospital stay, by virtue of his or her visiting privileges.

That voluntary hospitals in most large and even in smaller communities tend to compete vigorously has drawbacks in the proliferation of costly services. However, it also has advantages. Among the most important is the pressure on trustees, administrators, and the physician staff to seek out opportunities to strengthen and improve the services that their hospital offers.

Although prevailing high per diem costs have eroded the volume of free care provided by the voluntary hospitals (prior to World War II, charity covered, in the case of the best-endowed institutions, as much as 20 or 25 percent of their total expenditures), their continuing contributions to the care of the poor and the underserved are not inconsiderable, amounting to billions of dollars annually. Moreover, through their opportunities for cross-subsidization—that is, overcharging some payers to compensate for the underpayments or nonpayments of others—many hospitals are able to provide essential services to a large number of needy individuals, from the uninsured trauma patient to the premature, low-birth-weight newborn who requires many weeks of high-tech neonatal care.

Even more striking evidence of the critical contribution of most voluntary hospitals, especially in large urban communities, to the health of the uninsured and the poor is the substantial volume of service that they render in emergency rooms and clinics to indigent patients who present there, among other reasons, because most of the physicians who once practiced in their neighborhoods have relocated or died. The inner-city voluntary hospital has become the physician to the poor for routine medical care. Once again, a rational society would rely on a less expensive, more efficient system for general care. Until such a system is in place, however, voluntary hospitals will continue to perform a critically important function.

At the end of World War II and for the better part of a decade or more after, affluent individuals with difficult diagnostic problems or in need of tertiary care, that is, treatment of other than commonplace disease and surgery beyond relatively simple, standardized procedures, traveled substantial distances: in the Northeast from as far away as Maine to Boston; in the eleven southeastern states to North Carolina (Duke) or Baltimore (Johns Hopkins); in the midwestern states to Cleveland, St. Louis, or Rochester, Minnesota. These were some of the major regional medical centers capable of providing advanced tertiary care. Following the introduction of Medicare and Medicaid, the U.S. hospital system, and particularly the voluntary hospital sector, was rapidly upgraded so that a high proportion of community hospitals became capable of providing all but the most esoteric types of medical and surgical treatment for residents in their area. The costs of this transformation aside, the voluntarism that has historically characterized health care provision in the United States made it possible for many, if not all, citizens to benefit from an ever more sophisticated level of hospital care close to where they live.

The same voluntarism must be given much of the credit for the striking shift after 1980 of medical care to the outpatient setting, in particular the performance of surgery and advanced diagnostic procedures. More than half of all operations are now performed on an outpatient basis, and some observers estimate that the proportion will soon reach, if not exceed, the 75 percent mark.

In the mid-1970s, a group of entrepreneurial surgeons in the Southwest took the initiative of establishing and operating a for-profit ambulatory surgical facility. At the time, this innovative departure evoked serious question, if not criticism, related to safety, quality, "unfair competition" with local hospitals, and other related concerns. Time has proved the skeptics wrong. The leading voluntary hospitals have quickly or gradually followed in the footsteps of the innovators, and today a high proportion of their surgery is performed as an outpatient procedure, either at their main facility or at satellite sites. What started as nonhospital facilities for ambulatory surgery soon proliferated under competitive pressures into walk-in clinics, specialized diagnostic and therapeutic centers for oncologic, orthopedic, and rehabilitation services, and even comprehensive facilities that offer generalist and specialized care on an ambulatory basis to a wide spectrum of patients.

Some years ago, it was reported in the media that a patient 103 years of age had been operated on at the New York Hospital. The event caught the attention of the journalistic world because surgery on centenarians is the exception, not the rule. However, one of the major advances in therapeutic medicine has been its increasing capability to operate on individuals in their eighties and even in their nineties and as a result provide additional years of functional life. Before World War II, older persons who suffered a fractured hip were usually bedridden for the rest of their lives, often dying from pneumonia, for which there was then no effective treatment. Today, most patients with a hip injury can look forward to resuming their accustomed way of life within a few weeks, at most a few months, after a relatively brief hospital stay during which the defective hip is pinned or replaced. Elderly individuals disabled by arthritic erosion can be similarly restored to an active mobile life. The contributions of therapeutic medicine to improving the quality of life for the elderly have far outweighed its contributions to longevity. This appraisal was made as early as the 1960s by the late Walsh McDermott of Cornell University Medical College, a distinguished physician and medical educator. On the other hand, Lewis Thomas, another keen observer of modern medicine, also dismissed much of what modern medicine has to offer as "halfway technology." Unable to cure or to eliminate the causes of disease, the best that it can do (and often with limited success) is to moderate the adverse effects of disease and delay its fatal outcome. Before his recent death, however, Thomas is reputed to have become more respectful of halfway technologies.

Although many observers are disturbed by the uncritical commitment of most Americans to high technology, the vast majority of the public favors interventions that can extend their lives or improve their functioning (or both). The alternative, death at an earlier age, is a prospect most people do not find appealing. The American people may, in the future, reassess how much of the nation's annual product they are willing to devote to extending and enhancing the old age of the citizenry, but at present, such a reassessment is not high on the nation's agenda and it is not clear when or whether it will command serious attention and action.

Another source of strength of the American health care system is the fact that, notwithstanding the territorial expanse of the United States, its vast and diverse population distributed among fifty sovereign states, and its political structure in which the federal government's reach is constrained by the U.S. Constitution and other factors, there is a high level of uniformity and quality control over the many discrete institutions, professions and facilities involved in delivery of health care. Despite major differences among the nation's 126 medical schools in the resources available to them and in the goals that they have set themselves, all of their graduates must demonstrate mastery of the essential knowledge and techniques they need to undertake graduate medical education; on completion, most obtain certification from one of the twenty-three national specialty boards to practice in their respective specialties. Standardization and quality control of the medical educational system are all the more impressive when it is recalled that graduate medical education takes place in 1,200 different institutions.

Although the power to admit physicians to the practice of medicine is a state function, vested in the medical licensing board of each of the fifty states, there has been a remarkable degree of congruence in the standards that the state boards apply. This substantial uniformity is likely to be extended in the future with the implementation of a common national licensing examination. Even in the absence of a uniform examination, the state medical societies have exercised control over the entrance into practice of large numbers of physicians—immigrants and American citizens—who received their medical training abroad. Foreign medical graduates (now called international medical graduates) represent one-quarter of all active physicians in the United States. State policies governing their licensing vary considerably, but on the whole, the medical boards have dealt with this challenge reasonably, if not always equitably.

Although public policy and programmatic efforts in

the United States to improve the health of the nation
have been oriented to therapeutic rather than preventive
medicine, some significant gains have been made in
health education and health maintenance. Compared
with most other industrialized nations, the United States
has advanced the furthest in reducing the frequency of
smoking and the consumption of alcohol. It has also had
substantial success with respect to dietary modification
by the public to improve cholesterol levels, adoption of a
serious regimen of physical exercise, and the abandon-
ment of other suboptimal behavioral patterns in favor of
more salutary practices. These gains should not be ignored or minimized.

In terms of the health care system, the nation has
never faced up to the issue of providing all members of
the society with insurance coverage that would ensure
them access, or at least remove the financial barriers in
seeking access, to essential health care. Although the
issue has gained increasing visibility, the United States
has been slow to undertake such a commitment. There
is, however, another side to the coin: Americans have at
the same time refrained from decisions that would explicitly impose rationing, such as prevails in many other
advanced countries, where age and similar criteria arbitrarily limit the availability of high-cost medical interventions. Renal dialysis in Great Britain is a case in point.
Several months ago, a world-renowned American scien-
tist visiting the United Kingdom who was past the age of
eligibility for dialysis treatment, had to be treated sub
rosa by his colleagues who were determined to circum-
vent the regulations.

This is not to imply that rationing does not occur in
the United States. Money counts, often a great deal,

when it comes to deciding which patients receive open heart surgery, an organ transplant, or some other costly procedure. The important point, however, is that the United States has thus far avoided recourse to overt rationing as a method of controlling its outlays for health care services. Arguably, such avoidance is a failure, not an achievement, since distributive justice and equity might be better served by a formal system of rationing. However, many patients who would have been refused critical services under a formal rationing system have benefited from life-prolonging treatment under the more haphazard arrangements that continue to prevail in the United States.

Americans take pride in the fact that their society—including the health care system—is characterized by a pervasive pluralism. Government—federal, state, and local—does not dominate the economy, the educational system, or the health care delivery system. Most Americans oppose "big brother"; government should be guarded from dominating any critical aspect of their lives. There are advantages to pluralism—from stimulating innovation to avoiding the intrinsic rigidities of bureaucracy.

Nowhere else is this pluralism more evident than in the health care sector. The financing of health care is divided among government, private health insurance (employment-based benefit plans), and out-of-pocket payments by consumers. Philanthropy continues to have a modest role, particularly with respect to capital outlays for hospitals; it is also a residual payer for the poor. Pluralism in health care financing is vividly exemplified by the private health insurance sector: Approximately 1,500 private health insurance companies engage in underwriting health care coverage, reinsuring self-insured employers, and administering health care benefit plans for many employers who self-insure.

When it comes to the delivery of health services, specifically hospital care, the nation depends on three distinct types of acute care facilities—voluntary, public, and for-profit. Most major metropolitan areas of the United States contain more than one medical school and multiple teaching hospitals, with each institution investing a great deal of effort, energy, and revenue in seeking to establish, protect, and strengthen its unique position in the marketplace.

Clearly, pluralism is a two-edged sword, and although it encourages initiative, innovation, investment, and the rapid diffusion of new knowledge and techniques, it does so at a substantial cost. Nevertheless, in assessing the strengths of the current health care system, pluralism must be listed on the asset side of the ledger.

One of the striking advances in American medical practice has been a reconsideration of the physician-patient relationship and the evolution of new approaches aimed at engaging the patient in critical decision making regarding treatment. The physician no longer has the prerogative of instituting whatever procedure he or she deems best without prior consultation and discussion with the patient. Legislatures and the courts have established rules and regulations requiring physicians to explain to their patients the alternatives they face, particularly in the case of procedures posing substantial risk. Patients must be informed of their options and participate in the decision-making process throughout their treatment.

The first break in physician hegemony occurred

several decades ago with the establishment of federal regulations requiring biomedical research scientists to implement a formal system of obtaining consent from patients whom they wished to include in clinical studies. This was followed by the move to engage patients in decisions affecting their treatment. The most recent trend, which has gained widespread legislative and judicial support, is to extend to the patient (or the patient's surrogate) the prerogative of stating any preference regarding the initiation or maintenance of life-extending interventions in the presence of approaching death or irreversible loss of functionality. The patient who is the key party of interest may now decide on the application or termination of life supports, in direct contravention of the age-old medical ethic requiring the physician to do everything possible to avert the patient's death.

Even more important and more valued from the perspective of most patients is the freedom to change physicians at will. The vast majority of Americans who have good insurance are able to consult specialists for diagnostic assessment and treatment. True, this freedom is restricted in the case of individuals who are enrolled in health maintenance organizations (HMOs). Increasingly, though, even staff-model HMOs are providing point-of-service options, which permit the patient to go outside the established panel of physicians for specific treatment, although he or she must assume some part of the additional cost. The popularity of point of service underscores the importance that most Americans attach to freedom of choice.

Finally, the United States leads the world in biomedical research, with twenty or so major academic health centers at the forefront of scientific investigation and discovery. Moreover, the medical care system encourages the rapid diffusion of new knowledge and techniques to improve medical and surgical practice at home and abroad.

All of these distinctive strengths of the U.S. health care system must be incorporated and optimized in the inevitable structural reforms that will occur.

3

What's Wrong with the Health Care System?

In the crescendo of complaints and criticisms of the U.S. health care system, none is more frequent or more urgent than its skyrocketing costs. As a result of steadily rising health care costs, the principal payers are under severe financial stress that is compromising their ability to perform other critical functions. In the case of the federal government, health care outlays in 1993 will approximate $286 billion, or 19 percent of the federal budget. This figure does not take into account an additional contribution of about $70 billion by the federal government to the support of private health insurance through tax exemptions for health benefit payments allowed to both employers and employees by the Internal Revenue Service (IRS). With the federal government facing a deficit of around $300 billion in 1993, its mounting outlays for health care, together with Social Security, interest on the national debt, and defense (which is scheduled to decline), dominate the fiscal outlook in Washington.

The share that state and local governments assume of the national health bill is in the 14 percent range, amounting in 1992 to over $120 billion. Medicaid, a federal-state program to which the federal government contributes from 50 percent to 83 percent of program expenditures, depending on the state's per capita income (for the program as a whole the federal share is about 55 percent), has been growing rapidly. This is in consequence of the substantial rise in the number of persons with incomes below the poverty line and the growing numbers of persons over the age of seventy-five, more particularly over eighty-five, some one in four of whom require nursing home care. Over 50 percent of all nursing home costs are covered by Medicaid.

Most states report increasing financial difficulties stemming from their rising Medicaid outlays. The governors have noted repeatedly that escalating medical costs have left them with little or no scope to enlarge expenditures for urgent projects in other high-priority areas, such as education, highways, and prisons. Although the states have considerable discretion in determining the number of people to be covered by Medicaid and the range and depth of services that they provide, the program operates under federal statutes, which stipulate the categories of individuals for whom eligibility is mandatory and the minimum benefits that must be offered. Moreover, Congress has the authority to pass legislation mandating additional coverage with which the states must comply. Since the mid-1980s, Congress has taken this route to broaden access to Medicaid services for low-income pregnant women and young children. Although the governors have requested at least a temporary halt to further federal mandates, Congress has been unsympathetic because of its concern with the poor record of the United States in reducing its infant mortality rate, which far exceeds that of other advanced nations. Governors and state legislators see little prospect of escaping from the tightening financial squeeze resulting from their inability to constrain their rising Medicaid outlays.

The single largest nongovernmental source of funding for the U.S. health care system is private health insurance, primarily through the health care benefits that employers provide employees (and their dependents) supplemented by coverage that individuals purchase for themselves. In 1993, private health insurance accounted for almost 32 percent of total health care outlays, making it an approximately equal partner with the federal government. The employer community has become increasingly concerned with its failure to control steeply rising costs for health care benefits despite a wide range of efforts, from self-insurance to pressuring their employees to join a managed-care plan. Such prepaid, capitated plans guarantee their members a wide range of benefits, provided by a selected pool of physicians whose discretion in the treatment of their patients is regulated by the plan, and promises potentially lower costs than traditional indemnity coverage.

Many employers contend that their competitive position has been undermined as a result of their much higher health care costs compared to their foreign competitors, European or Japanese. But the issue of competitiveness aside, there is mounting evidence that growing numbers of employers—large, medium, and small—find the yearly increases in their health care benefit costs threatening to their continuing profitability.

The last major payment source is out-of-pocket expenditures by individuals for the health care services they obtain. Such payments cover just under a fifth of all health care costs, but only part of these outlays goes for physician or hospital care. Out-of-pocket spending is primarily for nursing home care, drugs, and dental care. Recently, the share of such payments has risen because of employer pressure on workers to assume a larger part of the costs of their health insurance coverage in the form of increased co-insurance and deductibles.

In addition to these mounting financial pressures on the principal payers for health care, the tenuous financial underpinnings of the system must be seen in the context of a second serious weakness: about 37 million persons lack private or public coverage completely, and perhaps an equal number have inadequate coverage. Moreover, private health insurance companies have pursued risk-management strategies that have made it increasingly difficult, or impossible, for many small employers to obtain health insurance for their workers or for workers to purchase it on their own, for reasons of price, occupational redlining, or refusal by the insurance companies to cover employees with preexisting medical conditions.

The reliance of the United States on private health insurance to provide coverage for most of the population below the age of sixty-five and the growing numbers of uninsured, underinsured, and uninsurable individuals constitute major faults in its health care financing and delivery system. It is one thing for an electorate to favor private over public health insurance. It is something else if, having decided in favor of private insurance, a substantial and growing number of persons are unable to obtain or maintain coverage because of market strategies that the insurance companies pursue.

Still another concern has recently come to the fore. Regularly employed members of the work force, many with good jobs and good benefits, who have been confident about the continuity and even improvement of their health care benefits, now feel threatened in view of the radical industry-wide personnel downsizing, the continuing efforts of employers to shift health care costs to employees, and the restrictive practices of private insurance companies. For the first time in forty years—that is, since the rapid post–World War II expansion of private health insurance—the capability of the private health insurance system to perform satisfactorily in the future is seriously in doubt. With premium costs rising at about 10 percent a year and wage and salary adjustments lagging far behind, the public is becoming increasingly restive about the availability, quality, and cost of health insurance that it has long taken for granted.

Other perceived sources of weakness in the health care system are reflected in the patent public resentment of the relentless increases in health care costs. Blame is assigned to the inefficiency of the hospital industry, the avariciousness of the pharmaceutical manufacturers, the greed of the medical profession, excessive administrative expenses, the overtreatment of moribund patients, malpractice litigation with its inflated awards, misused expensive technology, and widespread fraud and abuse by providers.

Further evidence of discontent and confusion among the public is found in their replies on opinion surveys indicating their desire for more and better health care services, which they believe the government should provide, but, at the same time, their reluctance to pay for these additional and improved services either out of pocket or through higher taxes because they believe they are already paying too much. The rescission in 1989 of the 1988 catastrophic care amendments to Medicare, which aimed to cover the costs of prolonged expensive treatment, was a dramatic case in point. For the first time in U.S. history, a significant expansion of social benefits was countermanded, in this case because of the opposition of the elderly who decided that the benefits were not worth the additional premiums and taxes that they entailed. The leaders of Congress and the American Association of Retired Persons who had lobbied for passage of the amendments were overwhelmed by the vehemence of the unexpected opposition.

There is a widespread conviction among professional and lay groups that the U.S. health care delivery system is unbalanced in terms of many of its basic resources: the number and specialty distribution of physicians, the number and level of sophistication of acute care hospitals, the utilization of high technology, and the number and types of organizational units involved in the financing and delivery of health care services.

Let us consider the shortcomings and failures that command broad, if not universal, agreement. Although most of the public are in favor of an ample supply of physicians (which the United States can claim, with 250 physicians per 100,000 population), there are serious problems in the training that physicians receive and distortions in their selections of fields and locations of subsequent practice. Approximately three of every four graduates of American medical schools become board eligible or board certified in a specialty or subspecialty after completing one or more graduate training programs. Although there are no objective criteria by which to determine the optimal distribution of the physician supply as between generalists and specialists, or the proportions of new graduates who should be trained in the various specialties, many leaders of the American medical profession contend that the trends are seriously skewed. Empiric evidence and clinical experience have been adduced in support of these judgments. In the first place, many specialists are unable to maintain a full-time practice limited exclusively to patients who require their specialized skills. The point is also made that an abundance of specialists leads to the frequent performance of diagnostic and therapeutic procedures in situations in which less intensive treatment would have been satisfactory. Finally, the overproduction of specialists, whose earnings amount on average to double or more those of generalists, has been an important factor in the inflation of medical costs.

The presumptive imbalance between generalists and specialists is a challenge that needs to be faced—the more so now that the locus of patient care is shifting from the inpatient services of acute care hospitals to ambulatory care sites. Since the acute care hospital is the principal training site for specialists and subspecialists, this shift has profound implications for the education and practice modes of future physicians.

A related issue is that notwithstanding the marked expansion in the physician supply, rural populations and low-income inner-city residents have encountered continuing difficulties in finding physicians willing to treat them. To obtain care, the underserved urban populations have turned to the emergency rooms and the clinics of neighborhood hospitals, where they receive episodic treatment by residents who are training in the various specialties; there is little or no opportunity for continuity of care, let alone the opportunity to establish an ongoing relationship with a physician. The conditions of practice and the earnings potential have been so unfavorable that most physicians trained in family practice, pediatrics, and internal medicine have avoided settling in areas where they could provide the rural and urban poor with ready access to generalist care. Although there is considerable disagreement about the optimal solution(s) for this non-match between patients and physicians, few question its existence and the need for early and effective action.

Just as the United States remedied the widely perceived shortages in the physician supply that demanded action in the early post–World War II decades, it succeeded in increasing the number of its acute care hospital beds and the sophistication of the services they were able to provide. Once again, however, the correction may have overshot the mark. The average occupancy of the nation's 5,100 acute care hospitals is not much above the 60 percent level; an 85 percent occupancy rate would be close to optimal. Since the recent trend toward ambulatory care will continue, the occupancy rate is likely to drop even further unless hospitals are downsized, merged, or closed.

The dominant factor in the economics of the acute care hospital is the disproportionate role of overhead—reflecting plant, technology, and trained personnel—in its total cost structure. Hence, underutilization, either of the individual hospital or of the hospital system as a whole, has adverse economic consequences for the society at large. Moreover, in the case of patients who undergo complex treatments in hospitals where such procedures are infrequently performed, effectiveness and outcomes are likely to be compromised. Many patients are not adequately informed about these risks and choose to be treated in hospitals close to their residence, by physicians familiar to them. The redundancy of acute care hospitals and of expensive, highly specialized services represents a double risk for the U.S. health care system: excessive costs and a suboptimal level of care to patients treated in hospitals that perform complex procedures infrequently because of low demand.

Closely related to the overcapacity of the acute care hospital system is the widespread diffusion of high technology, from magnetic resonance imaging to transplant surgery. There is no question that the availability of high-tech equipment and competent staff to utilize it have contributed substantially to improved patient treatment and outcomes. However, the rampant diffusion and duplication of sophisticated technology is not cost free. The economics of investment in high tech encourages not simply use but overuse. Selected studies suggest that overuse results not only in wasted dollars but often in hazards to the patient—occasionally even premature death. Except for a few states with rigorous certificate-of-need regulations, hospitals compete avidly in the acquisition and use of the latest technology. Although such competition has led to a steady upgrading of hospital care for the American people, it has its downside: excessive costs and the treatment of many patients in a suboptimal setting.

The vastness, the pioneering history, and the heterogeneity of the United States have resulted in a polity that is inherently skeptical and resistive of highly centralized forms of organization, production, and delivery of services and favors pluralistic arrangements. Hence, the health care sector confronts multiple sources of financing, alternative modes of delivering medical services, and a tripartite (public, voluntary, and for-profit) institutional structure.

A major concomitant of the nation's preference for pluralism in the financing and delivery of health care has been the elaboration of administrative and overhead structures to facilitate the sale of health insurance and the associated inundation of patients, insurers, and providers by paper that is generated in connection with the utilization of health care services. Here it is important to emphasize that physicians calculate their fees, for the most part, on a piecework basis—that is, by the units of service that they provide during an office visit. The same is true of hospital billings. A patient with an average length of stay (about seven days) is likely to receive a yard-long printout itemizing every intervention related to the hospitalization, from use of the operating room down to the aspirin tablets dispensed by the nurse in accordance with the physician's orders. Before a bill is paid by the reimbursing agent, it is often closely scrutinized and returned to the submitter with a request for additional information to justify specific items. This, in turn, necessitates further chart review and substantiation before payment is authorized.

The paper flow is only one aspect of a top-heavy administrative structure. Consider the 1,500 private health insurance companies that compete with one another in local, regional, and national markets. All of these companies are forced to devote sizable resources to selling contracts; moreover, most contracts must be renewed annually, and some more frequently. Germany, a country with universal health insurance, has a comparatively more segmented financing system—1,100 sickness funds for a population of 79 million. However, once an individual is enrolled in one of them, membership is for life.

There have been no definitive studies of the total

costs attributable, directly and indirectly, to our national predilection for an atomized, competitive health care system. The data that are available suggest that administrative costs in the United States far exceed those incurred by a publicly controlled and operated system, such as in Canada, or a quasi-socialized system, such as in Germany. To concretize the order of magnitude, a difference of just 3 percentage points in total overhead costs translates into "excess" expenditures in the United States of some $25 billion. Valued as pluralism may be, the American people pay a substantial price for it.

Closely implicated in the excessive paperwork are the elaborate and often duplicating regulatory bodies involving all three levels of government—federal, state, and local—as well as the large number of professional associations ranging from the Joint Commission on Accreditation of Healthcare Organizations to the residency review committees, each of which reexamines its residency programs on a three-year cycle. This means that a large teaching hospital with a range of residency programs is likely to have at least one group of visitors on site for many weeks over the course of a year, each looking at the same generic educational issues in addition to specialty-specific matters.

The past several decades have seen a proliferation of malpractice suits brought against physicians whose errors in diagnosis or treatment, in the view of patients and their legal counsel, have resulted in injury or loss of life. The increasing frequency of malpractice suits, most egregious in selected specialties such as obstetrics, orthopedics, and neurosurgery, has had serious consequences for both practitioners and patients. In the first place, the efficacy of the therapeutic process depends in no small measure on the mutual trust of physician and patient, a relationship that is difficult to establish and maintain in a litigious environment.

The annual costs of malpractice insurance in the most vulnerable specialties in selected states, specifically New York, Florida, and California, are often in the $150,000 range and represent a significant factor in the physician's cost structure. The most serious cost implications of malpractice suits, however, are not attributable to litigation but rather to the practice of defensive medicine by physicians.

All physicians, not only specialists and subspecialists, aware of the possibility of having to defend themselves against a prospective claim of inadequate treatment by a patient, perform a large number of tests and procedures not because they believe them to be necessary or desirable for effective treatment of the patient but because of the physician's potential vulnerability in a court of law should the patient's lawyer point out the failure to have undertaken a specific procedure. As in the case of administrative costs, there are no reliable data by which to quantify the waste incurred by defensive medicine. Several years ago, the AMA estimated an annual cost of $10 billion referable to defensive medicine. However, when questioned privately about their personal experience, a great number of physicians have stated that a realistic figure would be in the range of 15 percent of their total office costs. If correct, the AMA estimate would have to be multiplied five times.

Despite the extensive penetration of advanced communications technology in the U.S. economy, only modest use has been made thus far of the potential linkage of the many segments of the U.S. health care system through large, computerized clinical and financial information networks. The entrenched pluralism of the system has until recently prevented government or the private sector from undertaking aggressive leadership in the establishment of such networks. Some progress has been made at the hospital level, and there are various systems that tie office physicians to the hospital. Medicare intermediaries are gradually requiring hospitals and physicians to submit their claims for payment by electronic networks. However, progress has been relatively slow, and the volume of paper continues to rise.

The most serious shortcomings of the U.S. health care system relate to the lack of universal access to appropriate levels of care. For the most part, Medicare has accomplished the objective of the 1965 amendments to the Social Security Act: removal of the financial barriers that prevented many older persons from seeking needed treatment. The new payment systems that were established have enabled the elderly to obtain acute care services readily from both physicians and hospitals. On the other hand, the accompanying Medicaid legislation, which aimed to expand access of the poor and the near poor to the health care system, proved to be a more flawed effort. The legislation was restrictive from the outset by linking eligibility to prior enrollment in categorical public assistance programs, initially women and children on Aid to Families with Dependent Children and, later, persons receiving Supplementary Security Income. The states also had the option of including the medically indigent and recipients of general relief. By the mid-1970s Medicaid coverage of the poor reached its peak, with the enrollment of about 75 percent of all persons living below the federal poverty line. However, the predominant number of the southern states failed to raise sufficient funds of their own to draw down their full share of federal matching funds; in the case of states with the lowest per capita income, this meant the forfeiture of four federal dollars in consequence of their refusal to provide one additional state dollar. The primary explanation for this aberrant fiscal behavior was the disinclination of the dominant white taxpaying citizenry to raise additional state revenues for a program that would disproportionately benefit blacks. By the early 1980s, Medicaid coverage of the nation's poor had dropped from 75 percent to about 45 percent, although since then there has been a modest recovery as the result of actions mandated by Congress.

Another serious shortcoming of the Medicaid program, in contrast to Medicare, was the substantial difficulties of the urban poor in gaining access to mainstream physicians, those who provide office treatment to the majority of the insured population. Most state Medicaid programs failed to reimburse physicians on a scale commensurate with the federal government's reimbursement for Medicare patients. As a consequence, only a small percentage of medical practitioners in most large cities accept Medicaid patients.

In the late 1960s and the 1970s, there was a movement to fill this void with federally subsidized community health care centers capable of providing general medical care to the residents of low-income neighborhoods. However, the number of such centers was constrained, and the severe retrenchment in federal funding since the Reagan administration reduced access for the poor even more.

Although Medicare provides for the acute care services that the elderly require, it does not cover long-term care, in either nursing homes or at home. The only accommodation allowed by Congress has been to use Medicaid as a financing mechanism for long-term care for the indigent (elderly and nonelderly) or those who become indigent as a result of expenditures incurred through a lengthy period of nursing home care. In 1992, Medicaid payments for patients in nursing homes amounted to about $34.4 billion. This figure approximated 27 percent of all Medicaid outlays and over half of the nation's total expenditures for nursing home care. These means-tested benefits vary greatly by state. To many elderly and nonelderly Americans, the absence of insurance coverage for long-term care is a major deficiency in the U.S. health care system.

Let us focus on the elderly, who have disproportionate need for health care. Incontrovertibly, Medicare has greatly facilitated their access to services, in particular, to acute care hospital services. Evidence is mounting, however, that the ease of obtaining treatment has not been an unequivocal gain for them or for the larger society. As they approach the end of life, many elderly patients undergo heroic measures involving long stays in intensive care units and are kept alive by high technology even after their consciousness and functionality have been all but extinguished. Such terminal episodes often yield a final hospital bill of astronomical proportions.

The explanation for this frequently costly and inhumane treatment of terminally ill patients may be found in several interrelated and interacting factors: Americans have overestimated the capacity of high technology; responsible relatives are frequently unable or loath to provide clear directions to the physician in charge; the physician(s) and the hospital fear that if they fail to initiate treatment or they terminate it prematurely, they may be sued or exposed to adverse publicity. Aside from these billions of dollars spent, it is becoming clear to the public, legislatures, and the courts that individuals or their surrogates must be able to stipulate their preferences with respect to the initiation and termination of treatment. The indignity and the anguish of such futile treatment of the dying patient is an even more serious societal perversion than the financial costs.

One of the side effects of the preoccupation of the American people with the capabilities of high-tech medicine has been the neglect of the role that individuals can and must play in the maintenance of their own health through wholesome personal behavior and life-styles. The potential contribution that expanded efforts at preventive medicine and health education can make to the nation's health has also been neglected. Although there has been a marked decline in smoking and, to a lesser extent, the consumption of alcohol (largely among the better-educated, higher-income population), the nation has been plagued by increasing use of addictive drugs. There has also been a persistent underinvestment in prenatal services and sex education for large numbers of women, particularly poor young women, and in programs for adolescents and adults of both genders to prevent exposure to HIV infection and other sexually transmitted diseases.

The prevailing view of Americans is that if they become sick or injured, physicians and hospitals can restore them to health. Their own role in the maintenance of their health has been relegated to a secondary position; in many cases, health maintenance is not even recognized as a serious personal responsibility. The neglect, or at least undervaluation, of preventive medicine is best illustrated by the fact that until recently, neither private nor public health insurance (Medicare) reimbursed for such a critical preventive service as periodic mammograms for older women. Moreover, our society has been conspicuously remiss when it comes to ensuring that the immunization and vaccination protocols for infants and young children are effectively implemented. As a result, there have been recent outbreaks of measles and other childhood infectious diseases that a generation ago appeared to have been virtually eliminated.

Mental health is another arena that has not received the professional attention and resources it warrants. The generalist practitioner often fails to recognize symptoms of depression in patients and thus does not treat or monitor them appropriately. The toll in human misery, as well as in dollars (lost working time and productivity), is considerable.

The rapid deinstitutionalization of state mental hospital patients that began in the early 1960s has proved to be a seriously flawed policy based on a misreading of the earlier experience in Great Britain. It was compounded by the failure to anticipate the impediments to establishing adequate community facilities that would provide at least minimum support for discharged hospital patients. How did such a profound blunder occur? The psychiatric profession, politicians, and bureaucrats had become convinced of the benefits of deinstitutionalization. True, many chronic patients had been kept virtually untreated for years on the back wards of state hospitals. Nevertheless, it was an unjustified leap of faith to equate ineffective hospital treatment with the superiority of community care in the absence of postdischarge treatment facilities, to say nothing of adequate protective living arrangements. It is not surprising to find that most major urban centers are now confronted with large numbers of homeless people, about one in three of whom has a prior history of institutionalization in a mental hospital.

The growing concern with steeply rising health care expenditures has led to a focus on outcomes research: tracking the clinical status and quality of life of patients following a specific intervention, with the aim of determining the efficacy of various diagnostic and therapeutic procedures, especially those that carry a high price tag or are potentially hazardous. Outcomes studies are not easy to design, structure, or perform; nevertheless, there is early evidence to suggest that various widely used procedures are of dubious value, and even dysfunctional, for the health and well-being of many patients who undergo them. The protagonists of outcomes studies look to the translation of research findings into clinical guidelines that will alter physician practices and reduce, if not eliminate, the use of expensive and ineffective procedures. No sensible person would oppose the development of more and better information about the efficacy of medical and surgical interventions. And no sensible person would fail to approve the elimination of treatment modalities whose utility cannot be justified by careful retrospective assessment.

The current enthusiasm for outcomes studies, especially among the health services research community, must be tempered by the recognition that even in the face of countervailing data and professional judgment, many unproved practices and procedures continue to be performed with great frequency, demonstrating the intractability of habitual performance norms. Assuming that outcomes studies have the potential to improve the quality of physician care, it is problematic whether they will be able to make a significant impact on costs. In fact, such studies may paradoxically reinforce cost escalation. Higher costs may eventuate if studies reveal that many people fail to receive expensive types of care that would contribute significantly to an improvement in their health and productivity.

In considering the potential of outcomes research, it is important to remember that medical practice is and will remain an unquantifiable admixture of science and art. Although treatment protocols may prove useful and even cost saving in particular instances, they are unlikely to guide precisely the future practice of medicine, faced with the continuing rapid emergence of new knowledge and new applications, most of which has to be tried for a period of years before it can be evaluated.

Many of the weaknesses in the financing and delivery of health care have resulted in actions and reactions on the part of payers that have seriously disturbed the members of the medical profession by intruding on their clinical autonomy. Increasingly insurance carriers have required prior authorization by a nurse or some other nonphysician employed to interpret and enforce company protocols to admit a patient to a hospital and proceed with various tests and other interventions. All sorts of utilization review—preadmission, concurrent, and retrospective—have become the norm. The U.S. health care system is in danger of becoming gridlocked as physicians become increasingly disenchanted about and hostile to the mounting rules and regulations that payers impose on the deployment of their clinical skills.

The growing tendency of second-guessing the members of the medical profession is not the preferred way to balance dollar flows with medical outcomes. The achievement of significant gains in the nation's health that are the ultimate goal of reform will depend very much on preserving an optimal degree of discretion in clinical decision making for the practicing physician. There are better routes to effective cost control than arbitrarily subordinating physicians' professional judgments to the economy-driven decisions of lay payers.

4

How Did We Get Here?

Let us take as a starting point the year 1950, just five years after World War II, when the nation's transition from a wartime economy, politics, and social orientation to peacetime goals and objectives was well advanced.

The total health expenditures of the United States were slightly over $12 billion, or 4.5 percent of the GDP, just one percentage point higher than they had been in 1929, the end of the New Era. The small relative growth of health expenditures over this twenty-one-year period must be seen in historical context: From 1930 to 1940, the United States was caught in the most severe and longest depression in its history, and national income remained flat for an entire decade.

The period just prior to the entrance of the United States into World War II, the war years, and the immediate postwar decade constituted a major turning point in both the capabilities of medicine and the desire of the American public for broadened access to the health care system and its benefits. The first and perhaps the most potent development was the antibiotic revolution, which produced the sulfonamides, penicillin, and a succession of other wonder drugs that enabled physicians to bring under control most of the infectious diseases that had previously been endemic to large parts of the world or ravaged populations through periodic epidemics. Modern medicine was in position to make a rapid transition from what had been largely a "caring" function to one focused on "curing" patients. The surest evidence that medicine, prior to World War II, could do little more than tend to patients and alleviate pain is found in its cost structure. The per diem cost for a ward patient in a large teaching hospital in New York, Boston, or Chicago was about $5. Adjusted for the changed value of the dollar, the cost would be $50, as compared with current expenditures of approximately $1,000 per inpatient day at a major teaching hospital.

The new drugs were only one element in a much more extensive transformation. During the three and a half years that the United States was a belligerent in World War II, the medical departments of the Army and the Navy were able to make significant advances in surgery, the treatment of mental disease, and rehabilitation. In addition, the armed services led the way in designing and operating efficient evacuation and hospital systems, which enabled severely injured servicemen to be treated promptly and effectively by qualified specialists. The armed forces operated extensive ambulatory care facilities in the United States as well, which provided primary care not only to the servicemen but also to their dependents, thereby exposing millions of Americans for the first time in their lives to a well-functioning health and hospital system. This experience helped to fuel a much expanded demand by the public for improved access to health care once peace was restored.

Congress was quick to respond to this new demand of the public. It committed the federal government to major support for biomedical research, a commitment that rose steadily from $3 million ($30 million in constant dollars) in 1940 to over $11 billion in 1992. These research funds were aimed at extending scientific knowledge and finding cures for the leading causes of death in the United States: heart disease, cancer, and stroke.

The second seminal postwar departure was Congress's decision to make sizable funding available under the Hospital Survey and Construction Act of 1946 (the Hill-Burton Act), to assist states and localities in upgrading their aged and inadequate hospital plants. The construction of new facilities and the renovation and expansion of existing plants would provide many underserved Americans with improved access to hospital care and simultaneously facilitate their access to physicians who could be more readily recruited for practice with a hospital close by.

The war years brought health care within the reach of a large part of the civilian population too. Private health insurance grew rapidly once the War Labor Board determined in 1942 that trade unions could bargain with employers for health care benefits without violating the wage stabilization guidelines. At the same time, the IRS made a preliminary ruling, later permanently adopted, that such expenditures were tax exempt for both employer and employee. In 1993, these tax expenditure subsidies were estimated to cost the federal government about $70 billion.

The passage in 1944 of the GI Bill of Rights was the catalyst for the explosive rise in the number of young physicians who, on discharge from military service, were able to undertake or complete residency training so that they could (re)enter civilian practice as specialists. Although a number of factors were responsible for the widespread demand for specialty training, the fact that the armed services had granted higher rank, more desirable assignments, and more pay to specialists surely reinforced the decision of many veterans to seek specialty board certification.

Had it not been for the vehement opposition of the AMA, the immediate postwar period would have seen an additional initiative by the Congress: the provision of direct federal funding for the expansion of the physician supply. Such a recommendation had been made to President Truman by the National Health Assembly, which was convened in 1948 by the administrator of the Social Security administration, Oscar Ewing. The assembly reported that the nation had only 80 percent of the physicians that it needed to provide all Americans reasonable access to health care. However, the unyielding stance of the AMA deterred Congress from taking action.

In 1948 President Truman also lobbied strongly for the passage of a national health insurance bill. When it failed to elicit broad-based support, the proposal died. Despite nonaction by the Congress with respect to both issues, physician supply and national health insurance, World War II and its aftermath left their mark on the federal government. As the primary funder for biomedical R&D and as a significant contributor to hospital construction, the federal government was no longer an outsider to the operation and financing of the U.S. health care system, functions that had historically been relegated to the states and private philanthropy. In the early to mid-1960s its role would be further enlarged.

The third development that shaped the extant U.S.

health care system was the elaboration of private health insurance as the primary financing mechanism for health services for the American people. The United States may be said to have backed, almost by accident, into the prevailing system of private health insurance through the domestic vicissitudes of World War II. Hospital coverage expanded very rapidly in the postwar decades in response to advancing medical technology, the dominance of the acute care hospital in the provision of medical care, and the corresponding rapid increases in hospital costs. Private health insurance was extended to more and more of the employed population and their dependents, and the range and quality of the benefits improved markedly; by the mid-1960s, most workers were covered for extended hospital stays and for all physician expenditures connected with an episode of hospitalization.

Employment-based insurance, however, failed to meet the needs of growing numbers of Americans once they retired from the labor force. Advances in medical knowledge and technique made it possible for physicians to treat older persons for medical or surgical conditions that hitherto had been beyond their reach. However, since most retired workers no longer had insurance coverage, they were hard pressed to pay the steeply rising bills in the event of hospitalization. Moreover, their children, many recently married and with young families of their own, were generally unable to assume large financial obligations for their parents.

Even the conservative Republican administration of President Eisenhower sought to develop new federal-state programs that would be responsive to this growing national problem by expanding local welfare systems to cover the hospitalization needs of the medically needy.

These efforts fell far short; the programs were inadequate, and their linkage to the welfare system made them
unacceptable to most of the self-supporting elderly population. The Democrats took the lead in the 1960 presidential campaign to advocate a tax-supported social
insurance system that would cover the health and hospital expenditures of the elderly. However, the Kennedy
administration's proposal was rejected by a coalition of
conservative southern Democrats and Republicans who
voted solidly against it.

All of the concerned groups recognized that the problem would not resolve itself, and many, including the
AMA, set about developing alternative proposals to
thwart what they denounced as a giant step toward "socialized medicine." This proved a serendipitous boon to
the long-suppressed congressional effort to expand the
nation's physician resources. As the AMA concentrated
its lobbying energies in the early 1960s on the defeat of
Medicare, it retreated from its active oppositional stance
toward federal funding to expand the supply of physicians. Congress was finally free to act, and in 1963 it
passed initial legislation to provide direct support for
medical education. Previously, medical schools with large
R&D grants and contracts had been able to use federal
reimbursement for their overhead costs to help balance
their medical school budgets. After 1963 and especially
after the institution in 1971 of capitation payments as a
further incentive to expand their enrollments, the medical schools became the beneficiaries of increasing federal largesse. In 1965–1966, federal funds for research
and medical education accounted for about 55 percent of
all medical school revenues.

As the 1960s came to an end, Congress realized that

simply producing more physicians did not ensure that there would be a sufficient number of graduates available to treat the inhabitants of poor rural and urban areas that had long been avoided by physicians, no matter what their training (primary care or specialty), because of the adverse professional environment and the difficulty of making a satisfactory living. Accordingly, in 1970 Congress established the National Health Service Corps and appropriated funds for scholarship support to medical students in exchange for a period of committed service in a federally designated physician-shortage area on completion of their training. The following year Congress took the further step of putting federal dollars behind the financing of newly established family practice residencies in the hope that as more family practitioners were trained, groups that were on the periphery of the health care delivery system would have improved access to care.

There was considerable disagreement in informed circles, legislative and other, about the scale, scope, and nature of the physician shortage. Most leaders of the medical profession, including senior officials of the AMA, had by the end of the 1960s joined the advocates of an enlarged physician supply. In 1970, the Carnegie Commission on Higher Education, under the chairmanship of Clark Kerr, issued a report, *Higher Education and the Nation's Health: Policies for Medical and Dental Education*, recommending an increase of 52 percent in the annual number of medical school graduates in the United States. This conclusion was widely, though not universally, shared. In the view of the dissenters (I was one), although the physician-to-population ratio in 1960 of 142 per 100,000 was clearly insufficient and had to be expanded, caution had to be exercised to avoid too rapid or too large an increase. Arguing that most medical care costs are physician generated, the moderates saw potential dangers in creating an oversupply. They were skeptical of the contention of many medical economists that an oversupply would result in a reduction in physician fees and incomes and that there were no risks to the society from an abundance of physicians.

By 1973 senior officials in the U.S. Department of Health, Education and Welfare issued the first warnings of an impending physician surplus, and after considerable wrangling between the respective committees in the House and the Senate, a compromise health manpower bill was passed in 1976. The physician shortage was declared ended, and subsequently Congress began to withdraw federal funds for medical education, which had received priority over the preceding thirteen years (1963–1976).

In retrospect, it is clear that the single most important development to affect the U.S. health care system was the passage of Medicare and Medicaid in 1965 (Titles XVIII and XIX, Amendments to the Social Security Act). President Johnson's overwhelming popular and electoral victory over Senator Goldwater in the presidential election of 1964 gave him the political muscle to persuade Congress to enact Medicare as an entitlement program funded by tax dollars for virtually all individuals reaching the age of sixty-five. It was a two-part program: Medicare A covered inpatient care in an acute care hospital and was financed by joint employer-employee payroll taxes; Medicare B provided voluntary coverage for physician services financed by premium payments by Medicare beneficiaries and appropriations from general tax revenue. Almost everyone who was enrolled in Medicare A also elected coverage in Medicare B.

Unlike Medicare, which was wholly federally financed and administered, Medicaid was a joint federal-state program that sought to provide essential health care services to federally designated categories of the poor (welfare recipients), principally women and children. The states were granted considerable latitude to extend eligibility to groups that were not recipients of cash benefits but were deemed to be medically needy.

The legislative history of both programs is instructive. To the conservative medical establishment, the incursion of the federal government into any aspect of health care delivery implied the inevitable destruction of the independent, American system of medicine. A massive public relations campaign by the AMA invoked for the nation the specter of "socialized medicine" and "Bolshevism," and held Medicare at bay from 1961 to 1964. Ultimately, in 1965, Lyndon Johnson prevailed. Even then, the Ways and Means Committee of the House of Representatives (Wilbur Mills, chair) would not release the bills for a vote until the administration agreed to reimbursement formulas favored by the AMA and the American Hospital Association (AHA). President Johnson adopted a conciliatory posture and assured both the physician community and the hospital establishment that he did not contemplate any major changes in the ways in which health care services would be delivered to the American people. Physicians could continue to practice in a fee-for-service mode, and the federal government would determine their reimbursement rates using the CPR formula—fees that were customary, prevailing, and reasonable for their geographic area, field of specialization, skill, and experience. Hospitals would continue to be reimbursed on the basis of their costs. To underscore his good intentions, President Johnson designated individual Blue Cross–Blue Shield plans to act on behalf of the federal government as regional intermediaries in handling reimbursement claims of both hospitals and physicians.

In assuring physicians and hospitals that the preexisting structure of the health care system would remain intact except that henceforth most of the expenditures for the elderly and at least half of the expenditures for the eligible poor would be covered by the federal government, President Johnson and the architects of Medicare and Medicaid largely ignored the secondary consequences of the government's new role as a principal financer of health services. Over time, the federal government was to equal private insurance as a payer for health care; in 1992 each covered somewhat over 31 percent of the nation's total bill. Henceforth, the federal share will exceed that of employers and is projected to reach 34 percent in the year 2000 (assuming current trends).

Elmer Staats, Comptroller General of the United States at the time Medicare and Medicaid were enacted, was one of the few who perceived the fiscal implications of the newly passed legislation. He suspected that these entitlement programs would have far more profound consequences for the future budgets of the federal government than most legislative or administrative officials anticipated. That year, 1965, total outlays for all health care functions of the federal government, including the armed services, the Veterans Administration, the National Institutes of Health, the Indian Service, and other divisions of the Public Health Service, were $4.8 billion. The estimated total for 1993 came to $286 billion. Adjusted for inflation, this represents a twelvefold increase, reflecting primarily expenditures for Medicare and Medicaid.

Important as the new health legislation turned out to be in ratcheting up federal outlays for health care, it was far more important in transforming the decision-making and financing imperatives of the entire U.S. health care system. These have never been well understood by the public or the politicians, although they hold much of the explanation for the explosive cost increases that beleaguer the health care environment in 1994.

Some of the more important consequences that followed the implementation of Medicare and Medicaid in 1966 can be identified. Hospitals come first: Very soon hospital services accounted for the largest segment of national health care expenditures, roughly 40 percent of the total. By the time Medicare and Medicaid were enacted, third-party payments already covered 83 percent—five-sixths—of all hospital expenditures. However, the onerous task of raising the remaining sixth fell upon hospital trustees and administrators. To balance their budgets, most hospitals relied on a mixed strategy of extracting what they could from self-paying patients, cross-subsidizing services when they could, and depending on charitable contributions to cover the remainder.

The newly enacted Medicare and Medicaid legislation produced a major change in the financial circumstances of most hospitals. Third-party payments soon accounted for approximately 94 percent of all acute care hospital expenditures, and with most payers adopting the federal government's system of cost-based reimbursement, hospitals were assured that their future spending would be risk free; increased expenditures would be matched by increased reimbursements.

To concretize what happened: Prior to Medicare and Medicaid, many hospitals provided a considerable amount of care free of charge or below cost to both the elderly and the poor. With the passage of the new legislation, these groups were transformed from charity cases to paying patients. Prior to Medicare and Medicaid, most hospitals had to struggle to keep their operating budgets in balance, and their trustees were under even greater pressure when it came to capital investments, the money required for plant renovation, new construction, and the purchase of expensive equipment. Capital outlays presented a major challenge to most hospital boards, and in few hospitals did the physician staff obtain all the new technology for which they hungered. Administrators faced the difficult task of negotiating annually with the major clinical departments the list of purchases they would be permitted to make that year and what would have to be postponed for later acquisition. Even in the case of a major expansion, most hospitals encountered difficulty in borrowing money. In the late 1960s, borrowed funds accounted for no more than 30 percent of all capital projects.

The imperatives that governed hospital financing prior to Medicare and Medicaid can be formulated as follows: Most hospitals were responsible for the residual fraction of their expenditures that third-party payers did not cover. When large capital outlays were involved, they were seriously constrained because only a minority were in a position to borrow funds, and even those that could were obliged to raise in the form of equity much or most of the money required for any expansion or improvement. Clearly finances exercised a major constraint on the scale and scope of the capital projects that hospitals were able to undertake.

Medicare and Medicaid went far to change the role of finances. Once hospitals were convinced that third parties would reimburse them for whatever they spent, the preexisting constraints on their operating budgets were loosened, particularly the size of their work force and their salaries and wages, which accounted for two-thirds of the hospital's total budget. The new financial environment had an even more profound impact on capital planning and capital projects. Hospital financing suddenly became attractive to the private bond market. The hospital's accounts receivable could be used as collateral, and governments—federal, state, and local—often made direct grants in support of capital projects.

To increase the attractiveness of hospitals as borrowers, the federal and state governments put in place various arrangements that provided tax exemption for hospital bonds, a subsidy that further stimulated the market. Within a very few years, the hospital sector, which had always encountered difficulty in borrowing for capital projects, now faced the unprecedented situation of bankers' competing to become the lead house in issuing hospital bonds.

The large-scale redistribution of the American population during the post–World War II decades, from the cities to the suburbs and from the North to the South and the West, stimulated considerable new hospital construction. Nevertheless, many, if not most, suburban residents continued to rely for sophisticated care on hospitals in the central cities. Few observers anticipated in the mid-

1960s the sustained growth of suburban hospitals in the years that followed and the resultant decentralization of tertiary care. In retrospect, it is evident that the passage of Medicare and Medicaid greatly accelerated the preexistent forces that had stimulated the expansion of small community hospitals, the construction of new facilities, and the general upgrading of physical plant, technology, and staff. Many of these community hospitals became capable of providing a sophisticated level of care that could satisfactorily meet most of the needs of the local and surrounding population.

An important contributory factor to the improvement of the nation's hospital plant was the desire of most individuals to be hospitalized, when necessary, close to their home and family. This preference would not have prevailed, however, had it not been for the substantial increase in the number and types of specialists and subspecialists who, on completing their residency and fellowship training, had to decide on the location and mode of their future practice. The much-improved hospital facilities that were coming on stream in the suburban areas and in smaller cities convinced many physicians to bypass the traditional urban locations, already saturated or approaching saturation, and opt for open territory.

Here, too, the revolution in hospital financing was a potent factor. With ensured third-party revenues after the implementation of Medicare and Medicaid and money readily available for borrowing, community hospitals in the suburbs had little difficulty in obtaining financing for capital projects. With money no longer a barrier, convenience factors came to play a much larger role in the location, expansion, and upgrading of hospitals throughout the country.

To trace the full impact of Medicare and Medicaid on the nation's health care financing and delivery system, it is necessary to shift focus from the hospital to the physician. The relative shortage of physicians in the decades following World War II, specifically between 1945 and 1970, as a result of the rapid rise in the nation's population, the relatively constant output of the medical schools, and the increasing demand of the public for physician services, substantially reduced the amount of professional time and the volume of services that physicians had traditionally provided free of charge to indigent patients. An outstanding illustration of this change was the inability in the early 1960s of the Hospitals Department in New York City, the largest municipal hospital system in the nation, to continue to attract local practitioners for voluntary service on the attending staffs of its neighborhood hospitals. In the past, many physicians had sought these appointments, which carried with them considerable professional prestige. Viewed more pragmatically, an appointment to a public hospital was a potential source of patients whom physicians could continue to treat privately, for a fee, after their discharge from the hospital. In the tight physician market of the post–World War II years, however, most urban physicians no longer experienced any difficulty in maintaining a profitable office practice.

Community (voluntary) and particularly teaching hospitals were not affected to the same extent. Many physicians continued to volunteer considerable amounts of time on the wards and in the clinics of these institutions, where they treated large numbers of elderly and poor people who were unable to pay the (full) cost of their care. With the passage of the new legislation, charity care was for the most part an anachronism as the federal and state governments assumed financial responsibility for treatment of the elderly and those of the poor who were enrolled in Medicaid.

In the case of teaching hospitals, where medical school graduates obtain their residency training, the new Medicare financing arrangements permitted members of the teaching staff to bill for Medicare beneficiaries who had not been admitted by a private physician, and, further, the hospital could receive additional payment for both the direct and indirect expenses that it incurred in connection with the operation of its residency programs. The clearest evidence of this altered financing environment was the rapidly increasing stipends that hospitals were able and willing to pay to residents. Medicare made this flow of money possible.

Overstated, but only slightly, the introduction of Medicare and Medicaid fundamentally altered the parameters that had long determined the behavior of both hospitals and physicians. The key providers of health care services to the American people that had previously operated in a world of multiple financial constraints found themselves in an unprecedented situation in which the normal links between their health care operations and monetary resources had been severed. It took only six years, from 1966 to 1972, before Congress found it necessary to address the consequences and implications of its open-ended financing of Medicare. Some budgetary tightening was imposed as early as 1968 when Congress rescinded the 2 percent override originally included in its hospital reimbursement formula, and in 1971, as part of its national price control program, the Nixon administration set at least temporary limits on hospital and physician billings. Nevertheless, despite a succession of regulatory initiatives by the federal government, it would be fair to say that between 1966 and 1983, the year that Medicare replaced cost-based reimbursement for hospital care with a prospective payment system, the U.S. health care delivery system operated substantially free of financial constraints. In fact, the period could be extended to 1987, when the prospective payment system was implemented in full.

As for physician reimbursement, although periodic measures were tried by Congress and successive administrations to moderate rising expenditures under Medicare B, definitive fee and volume controls were not undertaken until 1992, when the Resource-Based Relative Value Scale (RBRVS) was introduced, essentially gearing physician payments to a time-effort index, replacing the previous customary, prevailing, and reasonable (CPR) standard. Moreover, Congress stipulated that in the event that physicians sought to enlarge their earnings by increasing the volume of services they provided, such additional expenditures would lead to a lower budgetary ceiling the next year. Full implementation of RBRVS is expected by 1996.

The operation of the U.S. health care system in the absence of significant financial controls from the mid-1960s to the mid-1980s goes a long way to explain the unprecedented tenfold increase in national health expenditures, from $42 billion in 1965 to $420 billion in 1985 (constant dollars). It would be difficult to identify any other major sector of the economy or the society, defense *not* excepted, in which neither the market nor governmental appropriations served as regulators. During these two critical decades, the health care system was driven by the decisions and wishes of providers and patients, with the required dollars readily forthcoming from the payers.

Starting in 1972 and continuing for most of the next two decades, the federal government, state governments, and employers engaged in a wide variety of efforts directed to containing health care costs, a goal that proved elusive. The federal government took the lead, followed by some states and a number of large employers, in designing and implementing a wide variety of experiments with a single objective: moderation of their health care expenditures.

The first major effort, in 1972, by the federal government beyond the initial price stabilization program of 1971 that was economy wide rather than health specific looked to the establishment of state professional standards review organizations, staffed by physicians, that would monitor hospital inpatient admissions under Medicare to ensure that the specific admission and the length of stay were medically justified. Since hospitals treating Medicare patients at that time were reimbursed by the federal government on a per diem cost basis, controlling admissions and expediting discharges seemed to be a promising mechanism for moderating hospital expenditures. A review several years later found that, however well intentioned the effort, there was little hard evidence of significant cost savings.

At the end of 1973, Congress, with the Democratic leadership in control, enacted legislation that made federal funding available for the establishment of new HMOs and the expansion of existing plans in the expectation that such prepaid capitated systems would provide more and better coverage at the same or a lower cost than the prevailing fee-for-service model. The Nixon administration had initially (1971) been attracted to this approach, but as the presidential election of 1972 neared, it was dissuaded from pursuing it aggressively by the strenuous opposition of the physician leadership. HMOs had had their start many decades earlier, principally on the West Coast, but their growth had been inhibited by the hostility of the organized physician and hospital sectors. Despite the willingness of Congress to provide federal funding for their expansion, the subsidy did not entice many newcomers. An important reason was the stipulation by the federal government of stringent conditions that the subsidized HMOs had to meet. Enrollment growth was so modest that the legislation was permitted to lapse at the end of the decade.

In 1974, the federal government undertook another legislative initiative, the Health Planning and Resource Development Act, an effort that involved the cooperation of the states. The federal government made funds available to the states to establish or expand area health services planning agencies, charged with screening and approving proposals by the voluntary and private sectors that contemplated new hospital construction, expansion of existing hospital facilities, or the acquisition of high-cost technology. The federal government stipulated that it would not authorize reimbursement for the treatment of Medicare patients who occupied new beds that had not been approved for construction under a certificate of need from the respective state's hospital planning authority.

Several years into the program, a review of the certificate-of-need effort could not demonstrate clearly and unequivocally that the substantial growth of administrative machinery and planning mechanisms had significantly inhibited the construction of unnecessary facilities and beds and the legislation was repealed. Although subsequent assessments were more favorable, the hospital and physician leadership had been soured by the cumbersome delays in obtaining approval for worthwhile, desirable projects, and this had created the momentum for rescission.

In 1977, the Carter administration conceived of a far more ambitious cost-control effort that aimed at limiting the annual flow of federal funds for hospitals to the regions and the states and lobbied hard for its passage. The legislation was defeated, however, as the result of a major campaign mounted by the AHA. The AHA emphasized the failure of earlier regulatory initiatives and recommended as its choice a voluntary effort by the hospitals to moderate their expenditures. Although the Carter proposal had passed the Senate, it was defeated in the House in favor of the AHA alternative. In 1978 and 1979 the voluntary-effort program produced some deceleration in hospital expenditures, but this was short-lived.

During the presidential campaign of 1980, the Republican candidate, Ronald Reagan, and his advisers extolled the advantages of the "competitive market," and for a brief period it seemed that the administration would introduce a radical new approach to health care financing based on deregulating the health care market. However, in the face of a rapidly worsening federal budgetary position, the administration opted for expenditure controls through cutbacks in Medicaid and in a variety of federal grant-in-aid programs to the states; the Medicare budget escaped with only minor damage.

It became increasingly evident to both Congress and the Republican administration that Medicare required fundamental alteration. In the fall of 1983, the prospective payment system was enacted, eliminating cost-based hospital reimbursement, which had been the practice of the federal government since the initiation of Medicare in 1966. During this seventeen-year period annual federal payments to hospitals had risen from $2.4 billion in 1967 (the first full year of Medicare operation) to $36.1 billion in 1983.

A review in 1989 of the financial effect of the prospective payment system by Louise Russell of the Brookings Institution, *Medicare's New Hospital Payment System: Is It Working?* estimated that the federal government had lessened its reimbursements to hospitals for inpatient care of Medicare beneficiaries by about $17 billion ($12 billion in 1980 dollars, or $18 billion in 1990 dollars) from what it would have spent under the preexisting cost-reimbursement system. Nevertheless, the total outlays for Medicare A (hospital care) and Medicare B (physician services) rose between 1983 and 1989 from $58.5 billion to $100.3 billion, and the resultant pressures led to the enactment in 1989 of a parallel reform, RBRVS, aimed at moderating outlays for physician reimbursement. Since fee and volume controls on physician services to Medicare patients will not be fully implemented until 1996, it is too early to assess their effectiveness. However, the following figures are relevant: Federal expenditures for Medicare B in 1990 amounted to $42.6 billion and are estimated to reach $50.9 billion for 1993. The combined outlays for Medicare (A and B) in the same years rose from $111 billion to $156 billion (estimated). Clearly federal cost-containment efforts have been playing catch-up, and they have not been successful.

The cost-containment efforts of the states have focused on Medicaid. Battered by federal cutbacks during the severe recession of 1981–1982, many states substantially reduced the numbers of poor people enrolled in Medicaid, and by the mid-1980s the program covered no more than 45 percent of all persons whose incomes were below the federal poverty line. Further, the states used their broadened administrative discretion over their respective Medicaid programs to realize other economies by restricting the types and volume of services provided.

A few states, primarily on the east coast from Maine to Maryland, continued to regulate hospital costs through programs that they had adopted earlier. A handful of the states sought and obtained waivers from the federal government permitting them to exercise control over reimbursements to hospitals by Medicare, which, combined with the states' statutory control over Medicaid and private insurance, consolidated their authority over virtually all hospital patient care revenues.

These efforts, however, failed to protect the states from the rapid upward drift of their health care expenditures, engendered primarily by mounting outlays for Medicaid, which were exacerbated after the mid-1980s as the result of successive congressional mandates requiring them to expand health care coverage for low-income pregnant women and their children. In 1985, the total outlays of the states for Medicaid came to $21 billion; by 1993 the figure was estimated to be $66 billion, an increase of 215 percent. Once again, cost-containment efforts, this time by the states, were playing catch-up.

This brings us to the third principal payer, employers, and their partners, the private health insurance companies, which provide underwriting and/or administrative services to the business community. By 1979, in response

to the implementation of the Employees Retirement Income Security Act (ERISA) of 1974, 7 percent of all
workers in medium- to large-sized firms (one-hundred
employees or more) received basic medical coverage
through self-insured health care plans developed by their
employers in the expectation that they would thereby
save money. In 1993, that figure was over 50 percent. It
became apparent, however, that although self-insurance
produced some savings, primarily by economizing in the
use of capital, corporate health benefit costs were continuing to rise very rapidly. Accordingly, business firms
explored a variety of other approaches.

Inasmuch as health benefit packages generally provided first-dollar coverage, the initial move of many employers was to introduce modest deductibles and co-
insurance, which employees, by and large, were willing
to accept, although in some cases the proposed cutbacks
in health care benefits precipitated a strike. Other employers decided to discontinue coverage for dependents
or, at least, to limit the costs or/and benefits for which
they would be responsible. It is critical to understand,
however, that these new financial arrangements accomplished little in the way of actual cost *saving*; they
amounted essentially to cost *shifting* by transferring part
of the cost burden from employer to employee.

Employers also attempted other strategies of cost reduction. Their early efforts, most of them dating to the
second half of the 1970s, can be classified under the
rubric of utilization review, which consisted essentially
of formal measures to intervene in clinical decisions involving hospitalization of an employee, the performance
of specific (high-cost) diagnostic and therapeutic procedures, and the length of hospital stay. In the case of

patients with high-cost illnesses, the employer might appoint a case manager, who would play an active role during the extended period of medical decision making.

In the early 1980s, finding that self-insurance and utilization review had failed to brake the rapid increases in their health benefit costs, many employers turned for relief to managed care. By encouraging the members of their workforce to enroll in an HMO or preferred provider organization (PPO), alternative prepaid systems in which hospitals and physicians offered the employer-purchaser discounts in return for increased patient referrals, employers hoped to cut their costs while maintaining the quality of health care services available to their workers. Over the decade, enrollments in HMOs and PPOs rose substantially, but the expansion was not reflected in any sustained, across-the-board moderation of employers' health benefit costs.

Disappointed by these outcomes, some large employers in the latter half of the 1980s, rather than shun the commercial underwriters, entered into collaborative efforts with selected major health insurance companies, establishing managed-care networks in which they and the insurer share the risks of coverage, and the costs to the employee are contained on condition that he or she agrees to seek treatment, when needed, from a panel of physicians and hospitals that has been preselected on the basis of providing good care at a discounted price. A subsequent innovation that has become popular is the option of the beneficiary at point of service to select a non-network provider so long as he or she is willing to absorb a penalty, often in the neighborhood of 20 percent of the cost.

It would be premature in 1993 to try to reach a definitive judgment about the potential of risk-sharing networks to make a significant dent in the steep upward trend of employer health care benefit costs. But in the light of the ever more vigorous efforts of employers over the preceding two decades to moderate their cost increases and the spotty results that they achieved, caution is indicated in anticipating that this round of employer initiatives will succeed. Why the odds may continue to be stacked against employers will soon become apparent.

A word about the strategy and tactics of private health insurance carriers in their pursuit of cost control is the starting point. Except for the recent initiatives of risk-sharing, managed-care contracts with large employers, the insurance industry has had little interest in cost control. The Blue Cross plans succeeded very early in obtaining discounts from hospitals based on the volume of admissions they covered and their record of prompt payment. The gains, however, were often dissipated by poor management practices and were not broadly reflected in lower rates to enrollees.   •

In recent decades, private health insurance companies have adopted aggressive risk-management strategies, aimed at avoiding coverage of individuals and groups that are potentially high users of health care services. Such strategies resulted in a decline in the number of persons with primary private health insurance coverage from a peak of 158 million in the late 1980s to 155 million in 1992, despite an estimated rise of 5 million in the total population. The concomitant increase in the number of uninsured persons, from 18 million in 1977 to 37 million today, can be laid largely at the door of the private insurance companies' risk-management strategies. Belatedly, the leadership of the insurance industry, federal and state legislatures, and the public at large have begun to realize that the United States cannot continue to rely on private health insurance for appropriate, adequate, and suitable coverage of the under–sixty-five employed population unless insurance companies are forced to provide policies at an affordable price to all employers and employees. To achieve such an outcome will require changes in regulation and the use of public and even private subsidies. These fundamental reforms are still to come. In the meantime, a substantial amount of cross-subsidization, especially for hospital care, continues to be practiced, so that patients with good private coverage pick up much of the health care costs of individuals with inadequate insurance or none.

We now have the explanation for the astronomic rise in total national health care costs since the passage of Medicare and Medicaid despite continuing braking efforts by the three principal payers. First, the introduction of Medicare and Medicaid effectively removed the historic constraints on hospital expenditures. Next, large numbers of the elderly and the poor who had previously been limited in their access to health care services could obtain care on the basis of entitlement or statutory mandate. Further, once third-party payers—in particular, governments—were picking up so much of the bill, physicians and the public came to adopt the view that every patient should have the benefit, regardless of cost, of all that medicine could offer.

The pre-1965 constraint of limited dollars on the volume and cost of health care services was gone. Although each of the three dominant payers has made repeated efforts to moderate its expenditures, each has failed. A major reason for the intractability of escalating health costs is the fact that no one payer, not even the federal government, has the ability on its own to reestablish or restore the classic control mechanism in which available dollars placed an upper bound on the demand for and availability of health services. The U.S. health care system broke loose from dollar controls in 1965 and has operated substantially free of financial discipline ever since.

5

Can the Health Care System Keep Functioning As It Is?

The devil's advocate would respond to the admittedly rhetorical question posed in the chapter title with a provocative, "Why not?" For almost half a century, since the end of World War II, the United States has introduced into the health care system only one major legislative reform: the passage of Medicare and Medicaid in 1965. This inertia speaks to the persistence of the status quo. Alternatively, the continuation of recent rates of spending for health care would entail demands on the principal payers that they might be unable or unwilling to meet. Specifically, the projected trillion dollars of additional spending on health care between 1995 and the year 2000 might not be forthcoming given the anticipated slow rate of growth of the American economy.

There is a second reason for querying whether the structure of the health care system can remain largely intact until the end of the decade. In addition to potential resistance from the payers, a loss of confidence by the users of the system because of the rising numbers of the uninsured and the underinsured, and the growing anxiety of many of the well insured about the precariousness of their coverage in the future could lead to voter insistence on early major health reforms.

In this chapter we will make a hard assessment of the likelihood that the principal payers will refuse to contribute the additional dollars necessary to maintain the existing system for the remainder of the 1990s. If these dollars cannot be extracted from those who must pay the bills, the issue is moot. Even if the funds were forthcoming, the pain and the resistance connected with their extraction would have to be considered. Financing issues aside, there are other sources of growing discontent among critical interest groups to suggest that the maintenance of the status quo is problematic.

It would be erroneous, however, to conclude that because the additional money required to maintain the current health care system between 1995 and 2000 may not be readily forthcoming, the derailment of the system (and its consequent restructuring) is inevitable. Powerful forces deeply embedded in the nation's ideology, history, and political structure suggest caution before adopting the derailment hypothesis.

One or another variant of national health insurance has periodically appeared on the nation's agenda ever since 1912 when Theodore Roosevelt, running for the presidency on the Bull Moose ticket, first incorporated it in his election platform. The proposal reappeared in the late 1940s, but once again it was given short shrift, even by the trade unions and other presumed friendly constituencies. In the mid-1970s, the chairman of the Ways and Means Committee of the House of Representatives, Al Ullman of Oregon, stated with assurance that Congress would pass a national health insurance plan and that in a presidential election year, the incumbent, President Gerald Ford, would not dare veto it. Moreover, his opponent, Governor Jimmy Carter, and the Democratic platform vigorously supported such a proposal. But once again, seasoned politicians were proved wrong.

The vicissitudes of successive attempts to enact national health insurance since early in the century were the result of powerful constraints on altering the financing and delivery of health care, which has historically been anchored in fee-for-service physician care and the dominance of voluntary hospitals. Admittedly, the health care system was substantially transformed following World War II by the rapid growth of private health insurance, with the encouragement of the federal government through major tax subvention. However, except for this indirect support, the federal government played no direct role in civilian health care until the passage of Medicare and Medicaid in 1965. It is important to recall that the passage of the new legislation was accompanied by assurances from both President Johnson and the Congress to the members of the medical profession and the leaders of the voluntary hospital sector that the new financing arrangements were intended solely to improve access to the extant system for two seriously disadvantaged groups, the elderly and the poor. All the other conditions of medical care delivery would remain, as they had been, under professional control and direction. The ideological pressures to contain and restrict the role of government in the U.S. health care system remain a powerful factor in the health care reform debate of the 1990s.

Several significant lessons can be inferred from the history of the World War II and postwar years. One is the alacrity, almost the eagerness, with which employers agreed to provide health insurance as a basic benefit for

their work force and their willingness until recently to
accede to continuous employee demands for more and
better health care benefits. It was not until the late 1970s
and, more particularly, the 1980s that business leaders
began to examine critically the financial consequences of
their supportive policy toward expanded health insurance benefits for their workers, as well as for themselves
and their management colleagues.

Little noted and less commented on were the attitudes and actions of the trade union membership and
their leaders, who were for the most part enthusiastic
about the steadily expanding health care benefits that
they were able to negotiate. A few trade union leaders
had identified national health insurance as a critical objective for the labor movement to pursue, but they were
in a distinct minority throughout the postwar decades.
Although the AFL-CIO supports major national health
reform, it is unclear where the nation's much-reduced
union membership stands on national health insurance
today.

In our federal-state system of government, residual
responsibility for providing health care services to the
uninsured and underinsured rests unequivocally with
state government. In the case of the categorical poor,
Congress reached a compromise in passing Medicaid: the
federal government became the principal payer, exceed-
ing the states' contribution by about 10 percentage points
(the ratio at present is 57 percent federal, 43 percent
state), while administrative control remained vested in
the states. At the beginning of the first Reagan administration, serious consideration was given to transferring
complete financial responsibility for Medicaid to the federal government in exchange for the states' assuming

responsibility for public assistance. The negotiations faltered, however, as the result of vehement opposition from the governors, who feared that this reallocation would prove disadvantageous to the states. It is evident that American ideology, history, and politics have operated in the past to keep the federal government at arm's length from broad decision-making power over the U.S. health care system. This triad must be factored into all assessments of a potential radical change in the status quo.

Other things being equal, the odds favor continuation of the current system of health care financing and the delivery of services in the United States, surely within the constrained time frame of this decade. Other things, however, are not equal, especially the total dollar amounts required to support the rising costs of the system and the disenchantment of growing numbers of the public with the future security and quality of their health insurance coverage.

Let us examine the projection that between the years 1995 and 2000 maintenance of the status quo might require the four payers to come up with a second trillion dollars over and above the $1 trillion in national health expenditures estimated for early 1995. The Congressional Budget Office in May 1993 postulated a significant deceleration in annual rates of increase from 11.4 percent in 1991 to 8.0 percent in 2000, bringing estimated outlays to $1.6 trillion at the century's end. Within these parameters, it will be useful to explore the alternative financial implications for the system as a whole and for each of the four payers should expenditures climb at their present rate to $2 trillion in 2000 or be constrained to $1.6 trillion.

From a national perspective, a potential reduction of

$400 billion over five years would amount to $80 billion annually. Substantial as this figure is, it would represent a savings of just 4 percent of the total projected bill of $2 trillion in 2000 based on the current rate of acceleration. In calculating the potential demand on the individual payers, we have assumed that their respective shares of total outlays will remain the same: federal government, 31 percent; employers and other private health insurance, 32 percent; state and local governments, 14 percent; and households, 24 percent (the sum exceeds 100 percent because of rounding). As its portion of a total "saving" of $400 billion during the last five years of the 1990s, the federal government could anticipate a reduction in its bill of $120 billion, or $24 billion annually for each of the five years. The simplest way of assessing this potential saving is to compare it with the total estimated federal medical payments between 1996 and 2000. Under a reasonably successful cost control program, the Congressional Budget Office projects that by 1995, the federal bill for health care will approximate $360 billion, rising to $583 billion at the end of the decade. Its putative savings would amount to about one-half of 1 percent of its five-year cumulative outlays and about 4 percent of its projected expenditures for the year 2000.

These figures suggest that Congress will not be catapulted into taking a lead role in the reform of the current health care system because of its inability to meet the steeply rising outlays that loom ahead. Staggering as the increased expenditures appear, they do not represent a significant factor in the current or prospective budgetary position of the federal government. Remember that the total deficit for fiscal year 1993 is estimated to be about $300 billion. An annual saving of $24 billion in federal health care outlays during the last five years of the decade is certainly attractive but will not by itself lead Congress to initiate a major overhaul of the extant system.

In assessing the prospective financial positions of the remaining three payers, it is important to emphasize that although each is capable of incurring varying amounts of debt, none of them has the wide discretion available to Congress of living on borrowed funds. It is this prerogative that has permitted the federal debt to shoot from under $1 trillion in 1981 to an estimated $4.4 trillion at the end of 1993.

Let us consider next the health care payments of business and individual purchasers of private health insurance, which together account for about 32 percent of the total, less than one percentage point higher than the share of the federal government. In the previous two decades, employers have directed increasing attention and effort to moderating their health care expenditures, so far with only modest success. We have identified the various strategies they have pursued: self-insurance; the institution of many different types of utilization review; efforts to constrain, if not cut back on, the continuing increases in the scope of their benefit package even at the risk of a strike; contract negotiations with employees under which the latter assume a share, or an increased share, of the cost of their health care benefits; and pressure on employees to enroll in HMOs, PPOs, or other managed-care networks that force their members to seek care from authorized providers and penalize them for obtaining treatment from non-network facilities and physicians.

The concern of employers with the remorseless increase in their health care premium costs and their diverse efforts to find ways of moderating them are pervasive. Since their outlays are approximately the same as those of the federal government (the differential is just 1 percentage point), it will not be necessary to repeat the detailed calculations of the potential savings to business from a reduction of $400 billion in the total national health care outlay in 2000. For employers, this would represent an overall savings of $128 billion, or about $26 billion annually for each of the five years.

What would this potential cumulative savings of $128 billion mean to employers? One gauge of its significance is the fact that in 1989, a boom year, total after-tax profits of all corporations amounted to only about $172 billion. In that year, their total payments for health care were equal to their total after-tax profits. The corporate sector clearly has a major stake in any broad-scale effort to moderate their health care expenditures.

The steep and continuing rise in employers' contributions to the financing of health care benefits for their current work force is by no means the only financial threat posed by mounting health care costs. We called attention earlier to the implications of their liabilities resulting from unfunded commitments for health care benefits to retired workers. Indicative of such pressures is the situation confronting many firms in basic manufacturing industries that have large numbers of retired workers with good health benefits and a much shrunken current work force consequent to their repositioning and downsizing. A major steel producer with a work force of about 28,000 faces the challenge of generating sufficient profits to cover health care benefits for these workers and their dependents, as well as for 70,000 retirees—about

160,000 persons in all. Each employed worker must generate sufficient profits so that the company can meet the health care costs of more than five additional persons.

Employers face still another difficulty fraught with dire financial consequences. Hospitals have traditionally resorted to cross-subsidization to pay for the sizable number of uninsured and underinsured persons whom they treat. Because of the history of underpayments by Medicaid and more recently by Medicare, hospitals have raised charges to private insurers to cover the category of "bad debts and charity." In New Jersey, where a statewide system of cross-subsidizing hospital expenditures in the inner cities has been in operation for many years, it is reported that employers and private insurance companies have paid a surplus charge of about 20 percent. Informal estimates suggest that most employers are paying bills between 20 and 30 percent higher than the costs generated by the beneficiaries for whom they are responsible.

Further, the vast majority of employers that provide health care benefits compete with others in their industry who do not and thus in effect enjoy a free ride. In the context of the increasing competitiveness in the global marketplace, many American employers contend that their ability to attract and retain customers is being seriously impaired by their health care costs, which far exceed those of their principal foreign competitors. This complaint has some validity; its magnitude, however, is largely or totally offset by the higher tax burden on their foreign competitors.

In sum, the financial pressures imposed by steeply rising health care outlays on the private sector will not result in the inability of most employers to meet these costs. Rather, the continuing upward spiral of health care outlays will be reflected in weakened balance sheets and a reduced capability to compete internationally.

This brings us to the third payer, state (and local) governments, which provide the nonfederal dollars required to fund the rapidly growing Medicaid program. In addition to Medicaid, state and local expenditures for health care services also include outlays for mental health, state hospital operations, and public health services. All told, the health outlays of state and local governments account for over 14 percent of the national total, considerably less than the shares of their partners— the federal government, private health insurance, and households. A reduction of $400 billion in national health care outlays in the second half of this decade would translate into a potential total saving for the states of $56 billion, or just over $11 billion annually. With annual state expenditures estimated to be in the trillion-dollar range in 1995, the potential annual saving of $11 billion in health outlays over the last five years of the decade would barely make a dent.

These calculations, however, do not reflect the full implications for the states of the future financing of health care expenditures. They are vulnerable to two contingencies at a minimum. First, state governments have residual responsibility for the provision of essential medical care to all of their population. Should the number of uninsured persons continue to rise in the future as a result of a cutback in the number of employers providing health care benefits for their workers, the states could be confronted with substantially enlarged expenditures for Medicaid.

A second challenge to the states is their ability to take

the initiative in designing a system of universal coverage for their residents. Hawaii, Massachusetts, Minnesota, Vermont, and some other states have passed legislation aimed at providing universal coverage. Hawaii's plan has been in operation for several decades, and the other states have programs in varying stages of implementation. The most recent and most ambitious plan, developed under the auspices of California's commissioner of insurance, specifies goals that extend beyond universal health care coverage to the integration of workers' compensation and automobile personal liability insurance with health insurance in the interest of administrative simplification and economy. Although the plan was developed and supported by representatives of many different constituencies, it has not been enacted into law. The governor vetoed the bill, presumptively because he was unwilling to run the risk of compromising the competitive ability of the state to attract new employers and retain existing ones in a deteriorating economic climate in which California's tax rates are considerably higher than those of neighboring states.

In the absence of major initiatives by the federal government to reform the financing and delivery of health care as promised by the President, the states will encounter difficulties in striking out on their own to develop plans for universal coverage and effective cost control. This dilutes even further the effect of potential savings between 1996 and 2000 of $11 billion annually in their Medicaid and related health outlays.

As for the fourth and last payer, households, currently a 24 percent partner in health care expenditures, their outlays fall into two categories: contributions that individuals make to the purchase of health insurance and out-of-pocket expenditures. The latter predominate. Out-of-pocket expenditures go in the first instance for dental care, drugs, and nursing home and home care and secondarily to payments to physicians and hospitals that are not covered by insurance.

Restraining total national expenditures to $1.6 trillion in the last five years of the decade would translate for households into a total saving of $120 billion, or $20 billion annually. The significance of the latter sum can be gauged by relating the estimated savings to the approximately $5 trillion of personal income projected for the year 2000. The potential annual savings of $20 billion amounts to four-tenths of 1 percent.

The triviality of this arithmetic result, however, conceals the seriousness of the concerns of many of the nation's 94 million households as they look ahead to their health care outlays. First, 37 million Americans lack health coverage of any kind, private or public, and about the same number of persons are inadequately insured. In California alone, over 6 million persons, one of every five residents, is uninsured.

Then there are many insured individuals who are locked into their present jobs because of the nonportability of their health care coverage. A potentially serious medical condition could deprive them of insurance coverage or place the cost of a new policy out of their reach should they seek other employment. Adverse trends in the labor market as the result of widespread downsizing, a chronic shortage of jobs (including service sector jobs), the loss in real earnings per hour and per week in most sectors of the economy over the past two decades, and still other developments are contributing to the anxieties of households regarding the future of their employment-based health insurance benefits. Their anxieties are intensified by the progressive deterioration in the health care benefit structure that has been noted: increasing cost sharing, restricted coverage for dependents, reductions in the coverage provided to retired workers, pressures to reduce freedom of provider choice, and the lack of coverage for long-term care.

Can the U.S. health care system continue to function as it has? A preliminary calculation suggests that the four principal payers are in fact capable of raising the necessary funds between the years 1995 and 2000 to permit the system to stay on its trajectory. Barring significant reform efforts aimed at reining in health care expenditures in the last half of the decade (or sooner), the incremental health care expenditures would amount to $400 billion over the final five years of the decade. This represents less than 5 percent of the estimated GDP of $8.6 trillion in the year 2000. Although failure to reduce total outlays for health care would place additional financial strain on each of the four principal payers, a successful reform effort will not be cost free. We must examine the costs of reform with greater specificity to assess how they may influence the future behavior of each of the key groups.

Several years ago, Dr. William Roper, head of the federal Health Care Financing Administration, pointed out that the serious imbalances in the federal budget militated against the enactment by Congress, even if it were favorably inclined, of any far-reaching proposal for health reform such as a Canadian-style national health insurance system, which would add several hundred billion dollars to the federal budget. President Clinton has turned this argument on its head by contending that major health reforms must be enacted promptly if the federal government is to make any progress in reducing its deficit and if all Americans are to be ensured access to essential health care services. However, the outlook for both action and outcome is uncertain since universal coverage and other improvements in the quantity and quality of health care services provided the American people will require more, not fewer, dollars.

Arguably, a major reform initiative led by the federal government would not necessarily result in a sizable increase in its own expenditures, but rather an enlargement and redistribution of the funds now contributed by the other payers. However, with each of the other payers avidly seeking financial relief, the prospect that the federal government would not confront a significantly enlarged bill may turn out to be unrealistic.

Evidence of the interaction between the unbalanced federal budget and health care reform is indicated by the long avoidance of action by Congress on the "play or pay" approach to universal coverage. Under "play or pay" it would be mandatory for employers to provide health insurance to all their employees. Alternatively, they would be taxed a fixed percentage of payroll costs to go into a national health insurance pool to cover uninsured individuals. The attraction of the proposal has been the promise of expanded coverage to most, if not all, of the uninsured, with little additional net cost to the federal government since most of the burden for coverage would devolve on employers that currently do not provide health benefits for their regular work force. There are, however, several serious, if not fatal, flaws in the proposal. The added costs might force many small employers out of business, thus increasing the number of unemployed and the number of uninsured. Moreover, by offering the option to "pay" rather than "play," the proposal could contribute to cannibalizing the existing private health insurance system if employers chose to terminate their coverage and pay the tax instead.

For many reasons, the employer community might be interested in unloading its heavy responsibilities as the principal provider of health insurance benefits for the under–sixty-five population. The time has long passed since the corporate sector was able to take the lead in putting a well-functioning system of private health insurance in place, overseeing its performance, and ensuring that it provided good coverage for most employed persons and their dependents at a sustainable cost. However, American business leaders have not put forward a clear-cut proposal to transfer responsibility for health care to either the federal government or a federal-state consortium. Clearly, under such a transfer, business would continue to pay its proportionate share of the required premiums.

The principal reasons that business leaders have not advanced a proposal for government to assume overall responsibility for health insurance are not hard to identify. To start with, although many industry leaders are frustrated by their inability to moderate their health care costs, they have no good reason to believe that shifting responsibility to government would necessarily slow the future increases in these costs, to which they would remain a principal contributor through the taxes they would pay. By retaining responsibility for covering their own workers, most employers believe that they will be in a better position to moderate future cost increases.

Consider further the many advantages that the ERISA legislation offers to employers that self-insure. They are exempted from state mandates with respect to the health benefits that they must provide; they are beyond the regulatory reach of state insurance commissioners and beyond the reach of the state tax authorities when it comes to health insurance taxes.

Aside from the specific advantages embedded in ERISA, most employers have historically aimed to keep government, especially the federal government, from becoming more directly involved in their labor relations and benefit systems. In their view, further governmental involvement would only complicate their relations with their employees and limit their managerial prerogatives. Turning to government to assume entire responsibility for the financing of the health care system carries a high, possibly a disproportionate, risk.

Finally, the goal of transferring full responsibility to government might prove illusory. The odds are that at best, a completely government-controlled health financing system could provide only basic health care services to the entire population. In that case, corporations that today provide a richer package of health care benefits would undoubtedly be confronted with demands from their workers for supplemental benefits at least equal to those they had enjoyed previously. Such benefits are viewed by many workers as an exchange for wage increases that they negotiated previously. Understandably, many employees consider their health benefits to be part of their earned compensation, not a voluntary contribution by their employer. To the extent that employers believe they will be unable to escape demands for supplementary health care benefits from their workers under a governmental financing system, they are likely to hesitate before supporting such a plan.

As one might expect, the governors of the fifty states have not found it easy to develop a joint plan for national health reform and to lobby for it. True, they have had some success (not as much as they would have liked) in prevailing upon the federal government to increase its flow of funds through disproportionate share and other adjustments to both Medicare and Medicaid, provisions that have made it easier for the states to cover incremental expenditures incurred in treating growing numbers of the poor and the uninsured. Medicare has also made it easier for hard-pressed rural hospitals and physicians to increase their revenues and earnings, thereby assisting them to continue serving the rural population.

A health care system that in a few years will consume from $1.6 trillion to $2 trillion is not a prospect that most governors anticipate with equanimity. Realizing that such an ominous prospect will seriously constrain their budgetary discretion, most governors would welcome the assumption by the federal government of responsibility for financing Medicaid, if not for all health care expenditures. The realists among them, however, see little likelihood that this will happen, in view of the tenuous state of the federal budget.

Given the diversity of their health care systems, their budgetary situations, and their political philosophies, it is unlikely that the governors of the different states will be able to formulate and undertake a broad program for health care reform that would engage the interest and support of the other three payers. However, they have good reason to believe that when a national reform effort is developed and enacted, they will almost certainly be key to its successful implementation. The vast size and the heterogeneity of the United States preclude the operation of an effective national health care system without the active and continuing cooperation of the states.

As for households, in a democracy in which every member of the body politic has a direct and continuing interest in matters affecting access to and payment for personal health care, the attitudes and voting behavior of the public are likely to be of primary importance in determining the scope, timing, and direction of major health care reforms. In the foreground is the plight of the 70 million uninsured and underinsured persons, along with the concern of increasing numbers of Americans because of the adverse trends in their health insurance coverage. The poor and the near-poor have seldom, if ever, had the political clout to impel the public and government to act on their behalf. If, however, increasing numbers of the middle class are at risk, or perceive that they are, as was the case during the Great Depression and the health care predicament of the elderly in the early 1960s, then corrective action is likely. The New Deal and the Great Society programs are proof of changes that can be made.

Although our calculations suggested that American households could absorb their share of even a $2 trillion outlay for health care in the year 2000, they confront what they perceive to be a losing battle for assured health insurance benefits and additional financial liabilities for their future health care. The likelihood that increasing numbers of voters will support a major health reform proposal that holds promise of providing universal access and cost control, and at the same time ensure them reasonable scope for choice of providers, is contingent upon their confidence that the proposed reform measure has a reasonable prospect of achieving these desired objectives. Whether the objectives are in fact realized will be known only after the reforms are implemented.

We are now on firmer ground in judging the ability of our health care system to continue as is. The answer is both yes and no: yes from the perspective of the financial capacities of the principal payers to cover a $2 trillion health care outlay in the year 2000, even though that figure would represent a doubling of 1995 expenditures; but no if the public recognizes that this outlay translates into an annual cost of $28,000 for a family of four. Moreover, the year 2000 has no special significance other than being the threshold of a new century. If the existing system continues to operate as it has, it will not be very long before the $2 trillion outlay will rise to $3 trillion, and the share of health care in the GDP will be heading toward 30 percent, twice its present level.

The financial capacities of the four payers, important as they are in assessing the potential of the system to continue functioning as it has, cannot determine the outcome. All that the projections can do is to suggest what may be possible, not what will occur. Although there are many reasons that employers have been reluctant to abandon their half-century-long commitment to providing health insurance benefits for workers and their dependents, the fact remains that the prospective steep increases in employer health benefit costs will eventuate in an almost certain rise in the number of uninsured persons, increased conflict between management and labor over cutbacks in health benefits, and an impediment to U.S. companies as they seek to strengthen their competitive position in the global marketplace.

Faced with the problems of deteriorating infrastructure, weaknesses in their educational systems, and deteriorating urban areas, which may well explode if left unaddressed, state governments have every reason to be concerned that a high proportion of all additional revenues that they will be able to extract from recalcitrant taxpayers will be preempted by the continuing growth in health care outlays. They will be ready to explore any reasonable alternative that holds promise of decelerating health care expenditures.

In the end, the 94 million households (read voters) will provide the definitive answer to the continuation of the present system, and that answer will be an unequivocal NO. The almost certain increase in the number of uninsured will be a potent factor, since the uninsured will consist increasingly not of the marginal poor or recent immigrants but of middle-class individuals, many with college degrees, who cannot obtain or buy insurance. Many others will be trapped in their jobs because of the uncertainty of retaining their health insurance coverage if they risk seeking other employment. And a growing number of households at the lower levels of the income distribution will face increasing erosion of their standard of living as the result of steadily rising out-of-pocket and total payments for health care.

Most important, the American people are close to concluding that their health care system is out of control, that it cannot correct itself, that none of the four payers acting alone can stabilize it, and that basic national health reforms are imperative.

6

What Can We Do About the Health Care System?

Agreed: The nation's health care system has operated under the momentum of expansionary forces set in motion after World War II that have now reached a point of no return, and rather than passively await the debacle as health care expenditures double every five years, it is incumbent upon the nation to reach an early consensus that the entrenched financing and delivery system must be altered and then to move intelligently and expeditiously to do so. This chapter focuses on strategic considerations that should help to inform the public, its many interest groups, and its leaders about the most urgent targets for change. At the same time it will identify issues that are not immediate priorities but may well invite action later.

Nothing is gained by minimizing the magnitude and complexity of the task of reforming the health care system. The difficulties of gaining agreement to change the course of the established system are suggested by the following pressures and counterpressures. Granted that the deceleration of expenditures for health care is the necessary condition that must inform all reform designs, the question immediately arises of the additional sources of revenue that will be required to provide every American statutory access to an agreed-upon level of essential care. The approach to a program for reform put forth here is predicated on the prompt moderation of the rate of increase in health care expenditures, not a reduction in total spending. Although providing coverage for the uninsured will not be simple, sound fiscal analyses and projections indicate that the incremental costs of statutory coverage for all do not present a major stumbling block. The net additional cost has been estimated to be around $50 billion annually, or about 5.5 percent of estimated total outlays for 1993. It may be useful to recall that during the preceding five years, 1987–1992, the annual rate of increase in total expenditures averaged 10 percent.

Providing coverage for the uninsured appears to be a potentially less costly undertaking than many people believe, and it can be accomplished within a broader reform effort aimed at slowing future total outlays for health care. Consider, nevertheless, the stresses and strains that universal coverage within a constrained expenditure target would impose on the majority of Americans with good health insurance who have been accustomed to the benefits of an ever more sophisticated system of health care delivery. Fueled by the large outlays of new dollars, these benefits translated into an increased quantity and quality of health care services available to those with coverage, which contributed to the prolongation of their lives, reduction in pain and disability, and increased functionality, especially in their later years. Is it not inevitable that with rigorous control over the new dollars flowing into the health care system, the American people will have reduced access to medical advances both because of a slowed rate of innovation and financial barriers to utilization?

This is a crucial question—probably the most crucial—if a case is to be made for early and fundamental reforms aimed at moderating the rate at which new resources are made available to the health care system. Three answers are possible, and each should be examined. The first, on the whole assumed but occasionally supported by argument, is that the existing system should not be altered, and no effort should be made to institute a system of global budgeting designed to limit the inflow of resources, for the simple reason that the benefits to the public from the present uncontrolled funding exceed any alternative, including global budgeting. Although many advocates of the status quo would agree that consumption by the health sector of an ever larger proportion of the nation's output of goods and services cannot continue indefinitely, they see no reason to intervene now. Only if the system fails eventually to correct itself would intervention be necessary. Between now and then, however, much can happen, and it is better to avoid premature actions that might jeopardize much that is valuable for the sake of putative, but unproved and unprovable, gains.

The second answer is that the resources available now to the health care system are ample to provide both a desirable level of coverage for all and to pay for the advances that will be produced by continuing research and technological development if only the "waste" in the system were eliminated and the recaptured resources diverted to these goals. Since the redistribution-of-existing-resources approach to moderating the rate of health care spending has gained wide currency, the arguments advanced in its support deserve serious inspection. They will be considered sequentially on a continuum from the least disruptive of the status quo to the most radical.

The accumulation in recent years of large bodies of data on the utilization of hospital services has encouraged health policy analysts and leaders of clinical research to review retrospectively the efficacy of various commonly performed interventions, in particular high-cost diagnostic and surgical procedures. In the case of some procedures, outcomes studies have found that a large number of patients, sometimes as many as one-third, failed to profit, and for many others, their appropriateness was questionable. These outcomes studies are aimed at the development of clinical criteria to guide physician practices in the future, particularly in the surgical arena. The conclusions and the potential utility of such studies have been sufficiently persuasive that Congress now appropriates over $100 million annually for the support of this effort in the expectation of substantial savings in dollars and gains in quality of care. Dr. Robert H. Brook of the University of California, Los Angeles, and RAND, a pioneer in outcomes research, has cautioned, however, that although more resources dedicated to such studies will add to the safety and efficacy of many new interventions, potential large savings are problematic, since the studies may reveal that the number of patients who undergo unneeded or counterindicated services is offset by the number of others for whom the particular procedures would be beneficial but who have thus far not received them because of physician caution, lack of hospital resources, and other reasons. From the record to date, it is unclear that outcomes studies will lead to a significant recapture of scarce health resources.

Another approach, favored by both the AMA and President Clinton, is the reform of the tort system used to recover damages as the result of physician malpractice. Although malpractice insurance is estimated to cost as much as $8 billion annually, the presumption among analysts is that this figure accounts for only a small part of the total costs generated by the practice of defensive medicine, which may be five times larger or more. A number of state legislatures have acted in recent years to limit the dollar amount of damages that a plaintiff can recover, in particular for "pain and suffering." Although there are doubtless many opportunities to reform malpractice procedures with an aim of compensating the injured more equitably and promptly and at the same time contributing to an improved quality of care, there is little reason to expect that even a radically reformed system will recapture a substantial amount of current resources for effective redeployment.

Since the beginning of the 1970s when Dr. Paul Ellwood, the director of InterStudy, a distinguished policy analysis center, succeeded in persuading President Nixon of the cost-saving potential of prepaid health care plans, which he renamed health maintenance organizations, the proposition has been dangled before the American people that if they would shift their allegiance from physicians in private fee-for-service practice to prepaid, capitated plans, their health care expenditures (and those of their employer and the government) could be substantially reduced. At the same time, they would be assured of more comprehensive health care, including preventive services. Although Congress made federal funds available in 1973 to speed the growth of HMO enrollment, it was not until the 1980s that HMOs and their offshoots—preferred provider organizations and related types of capitated or managed-care plans—began to expand rapidly. Managed-care enrollment in 1993 was approximately 43 million (17percent of all Americans and 20 percent of the insured population), of which Kaiser-Permanente, the California archetype, accounted for about 6.6 million.

Students of health care delivery systems who have examined the relative costs and quality of health care provided by well-managed HMOs and by the fee-for-service sector have found a considerable cost advantage (10 percent or more) in the former, largely as the result of their lower rate of hospital admissions and their constraints on the utilization of specialist services. The spurt in HMO enrollments that occurred in the 1980s reflected principally the expansion of independent practice associations, a variant of the HMO mode, in which private practitioners agree to treat enrollees for a stipulated (discounted) fee and to comply with practice regulations specified by the HMO. The decline during the 1980s in overall patient admissions and patient days in acute care hospitals, however, reduced, if it did not eliminate, a principal cost advantage of HMOs.

Many employers enlisted both persuasion and dollar incentives in the 1980s to encourage the enrollment of their employees in HMOs, and their success was reflected in the substantial membership growth of prepayment plans. However, the expected deceleration in employers' health care costs proved disappointing. Currently employers are attracted to a newer variant of the HMO: risk-sharing arrangements with large insurance companies that contract to provide a selected network of physicians and hospitals committed to performing quality care efficiently and economically. It remains to be seen whether this version of managed care will be more effective than its predecessors in moderating employers' cost increases. In sum, the long-heralded economies of managed care, first enunciated by Paul Ellwood in 1970, elaborated by Professor Alain Enthoven of Stanford University in 1977, and repeatedly touted since then, have yet to be demonstrated. Inasmuch as most physicians have until recently avoided practicing as members of an HMO, the rapidity and the extent to which the promise of this alternative delivery system materializes is problematic.

Some critics contend that the U.S. commitment of the overwhelming proportion of its health dollars to acute care services is a serious misallocation of health resources. The system, it is argued, overinvests in efforts to prolong the lives of patients as they approach death and underinvests in prevention and health education, where additional dollars would have much larger payoffs. The paucity of resources directed to preventive and health educational activities is trenchantly evident in the large numbers of teenage pregnancies and births to pregnant women who fail to receive reproductive and prenatal care.

Without contesting the fact that the U.S. health system is skewed toward acute care, it is unclear how much scope there is for recovering sizable resources by program redirection. A significant reduction of the hospitalization rates of Medicare patients would require restricting the use of specific procedures and treatments by arbitrary criteria such as age or physical status, and such explicit rationing, though prevalent in Great Britain, is unlikely to win approval in the United States.

The heroic treatment of dying patients is something else. Here there are opportunities for both humanitarian and economic gains. In fact, with a strong assist from the courts, the American public is gradually taking up the option of specifying in advance or at the time of hospital admission whether they wish to be subjected to heroic terminal treatments. The proliferation of living wills and the authorization of relatives or close friends to act as surrogates and refuse life-prolonging measures on their behalf reflect the growing sensitivity of individuals to the limitations and often the futility of medical treatment during the final weeks and days of life.

Efforts directed toward prevention and health education are eminently desirable, but it is doubtful that they will produce significant resource savings in the short and middle term. The many impressive cost-benefit ratios that have gained wide currency, such as one dollar spent for prenatal care saves three dollars in expenditures for neonatal care, must be looked at critically. No one questions the importance of making prenatal care readily available to all women during the first trimester of pregnancy. It does not follow, however, that failure of many to obtain care is necessarily attributable to lack of access. In many cases, pregnant women are reluctant to seek care knowing that the physician whom they see will try seriously to persuade them to stop smoking, drinking, and using addictive drugs, all of which pose high risks to their baby.

Similarly, most Americans are aware of the importance of a low-fat diet, regular physical exercise, adequate sleep, and other good health habits. But given the pres-

sures of daily life, high levels of tension, and the tendency to disregard the future consequences of their
actions, many are unable to alter their behavior in ways
that would contribute positively to their health.

Savings in resource allocation undoubtedly could be
achieved if people actually followed these desirable reg-
imens. However, it is questionable that vigorous implementation is a realistic goal, and without it, there would
be little yield of "saved" resources to underwrite the
continuing new treatment modalities spawned by medical progress.

Closely related to the approach of realizing potential
savings through changes in clinical practice and personal
behavior is the rationing of medical services. Rationing
seeks to achieve a better balance between scarce resources and optimal utilization by denying certain costly
services to specific categories of patients defined by age,
gender, race, payment status, potential productivity, or
other criteria. It is obvious that there has always been
implicit rationing of medical care based on the availability of resources. Cardiac patients admitted to a small rural
hospital do not receive the range and intensity of services
that are provided in a major teaching hospital. But this is
not what is implied by the term *rationing*. Rationing re-
fers to agreed-to cutoff points in the range and quality of
treatments, primarily high-cost treatments, that will be
made available to different categories of patients, all of
whom could profit in varying degrees from such procedures. In order to reduce the total outlays of the health
care system, only designated groups of patients will receive the specified procedures. The outstanding effort
along this line is the recently approved legislation by the
state of Oregon to implement a priority listing of the

services that will be provided to Medicaid patients. By setting a predetermined cutoff point for specific services available under Medicaid, the state anticipates that it will be able to provide more effective care to all of the poor. Although the Oregon plan has been criticized because of the criteria used in its ranking of approved services, there is little doubt that the rationing system now being followed is likely to lead to a "bigger bang for the buck." More of the poor will have access to essential services. But as in the case of the elderly under Medicare, overt rationing does not appear to be a socially acceptable mechanism for a significant redistribution of health resources.

By far the most ambitious and most debated of the various strategies to optimize the use of current resources is administrative reform, specifically the elimination of private health insurance and the adoption of a single-payer system. The prototype is the governmental health financing system that operates in Canada. The proponents of a Canadian-type plan for the United States have estimated a significant savings in our health care expenditures if we were to rely on government—federal, state, or both—as the sole payer and withdraw the plethora of private insurance companies from the health financing market. Although there is no agreement among the experts, calculations of the potential savings that would accrue from replicating the Canadian approach in the United States are on the order of 10 percent. If valid, upwards of $90 billion might be freed through administrative reform for reinvestment in the health care system.

For all its presumed advantages, the Canadian experience does not appear to be a usable model for the United States. First, its major attributes—universal coverage and the reduction of administrative costs—would, if introduced in the United States, result ineluctably in increased total expenditures. Reliable estimates, based on 1991 data, indicate that the cost of expanded utilization of health services would exceed administrative savings by over $30 billion, an increase that the U.S. health care system could absorb, but only with difficulty, in a cost-containment environment. Second, there is nothing in recent U.S. political, social, or economic policy to suggest that the nation is ready to consider, much less to act upon, the elimination of the role of the private insurance industry in the future financing of U.S. health care. It is important to recall that currently the contribution of private insurance to total health care financing equals that of the federal government.

The third barrier to adopting the Canadian model is by all odds the most powerful: Americans do not believe that the centralization in government of all decision-making power over financing the operations of the health care system as well as future capital investments is desirable. Historically, Canadians have demonstrated a confidence in the capacity of their government to respond to the essential needs of the citizenry. Americans, in contrast, have a critical, even cynical, view of the capability of government to manage even relatively simple functions like the postal system, much less something as complex as financing health care services for the entire population. The preference for private initiative and, at most, limited interference by government are dominant values in American society. It is also well to remember that the U.S. population is ten times as large as Canada's and far more diverse.

It would be difficult, and probably not rewarding, to

explore the relative dollar costs of providing the equivalent quantity and quality of medical services in Canada and in the United States. A careful reading of the analyses that have been published points up a great many technical difficulties in identifying and developing the appropriate data sets needed to make valid comparisons. However, most, if not all, analysts would agree to the following general assessment: Although the Canadian ratio of per capita health care spending to GDP is several percentage points below, and its administrative costs considerably below, those of the United States, the acceleration in its total expenditures in recent years has approximated, if not outpaced, that of the United States. Further, there is controversy among analysts with respect to the quality implications of Canada's heavy reliance on general practitioners, the lower technological sophistication of its hospitals, and the longer waiting times for elective surgery. Are these major or minor, negative or positive factors when comparing the relative quality of the care provided the average citizen by the two systems?

In terms of the potential recapture of some part of the resources currently invested by the United States in its health care delivery system, the experience of our northern neighbor offers at least one useful clue: It should be possible to make significant economies over time in reducing the high administrative costs embedded in our free-wheeling system of multiple sellers of private health insurance, multiple providers of care, and multiple intermediaries, all engaged in mountainous record keeping.

Although there is a potential for savings in many sectors of the U.S. health care system, clearly there is little reason to believe that they can be achieved rapidly, if at all. It follows that the ominous trend of escalating health care expenditures for the remainder of this decade cannot be financed to any significant degree by reallocating resources that are currently deployed. Such resources must be recaptured before they can be redeployed, and their recapture is problematic. That being the case, the primary focus of U.S. health policy must be on moderating the rate at which additional resources are permitted to flow into the system. Suggestions for the steps required to achieve a significant moderation in the nation's health care expenditures are elaborated in chapters 9 and 10. In the remainder of this chapter, we will examine the professional, economic, and institutional realities that set the bounds within which any health care delivery system must perform. These realities must be kept in the forefront of any effort aimed at slowing the inflow of new dollars into the system.

The dramatic successes of clinical medicine since World War II have been grounded in the sizable, continuing investments that the United States has made to support an ever larger biomedical R&D effort. Although no one can foretell what the new molecular biology and biotechnology will contribute to the advancement of medicine, there are good reasons for optimism about the gains that lie ahead. Even in the face of uncertainty as to when, if ever, we will gain control over cancer, Alzheimer's disease, AIDS, and many other pathologies, it would make little or no sense for the United States to cut back on an R&D effort that currently consumes around 3 percent of our health care budget. Many argue that the research effort should be expanded; few recommend that it be cut back.

The future financing of R&D becomes more problematic when attention shifts from research to development, and the question is raised of the consequences of decelerating future dollar inflows into the health care system. Prior to the enactment of Medicare in 1965, the rate of dissemination of new technology was contingent upon the ability and willingness of hospital trustees to raise the capital funds needed for its purchase and to budget for the increased operating expenses that the new services entailed. These constraints were removed when the federal government decided to join the other payers to reimburse hospitals on the basis of cost, a decision that led to a rapid diffusion of increasingly expensive devices and services. Federal and state governments made periodic efforts to limit the adoption of new technology, but for the most part they were unsuccessful. Control of total health care expenditures in the future will have to deal with the issue of the continuous acquisition of marginally improved technology and the unnecessary duplication of valuable but expensive new equipment and services by institutions in the same or adjacent areas.

The second, and overarching, consideration in any serious effort to slow national health care expenditures is the strategic role of physicians and their preferred ways of practicing medicine. Cost-containment attempts by both the federal government and employers during the past two decades have led to a large number of rules and regulations aimed at restricting the independent exercise of clinical judgment by physicians in treating their patients. Second-guessing physicians has become the preferred tactic of payers to constrain outlays. This system does not reflect primarily an adversarial attitude of government and corporate management to the medical profession, but rather the growing awareness of payers that in a fee-for-service, essentially piecework mode of practice, some limitations must be placed on the freedom of physicians to undertake their preferred treatment of patients with no regard to the payment for their care. However, determinations of medical treatment based on insurers' or payers' protocols, as interpreted by nurses at the end of a telephone line, are far from the mechanism of choice for the parties involved—payers, physicians, and patients.

One of the imperatives of a reform approach aimed at moderating total dollar outlays must be to design an optimal structure that will allow physicians maximum leeway to exercise their clinical judgment within a set of total resource constraints. The serious shortfall in the recent past in balancing these conflicting objectives must serve as a warning. An approach is needed that is responsive to these financial constraints without undermining the standards and morale of the medical profession.

In this connection, it is worth noting that U.S. health care policy has not paid sufficient attention to the impact of the numbers, fields of specialization, and practice locations of physicians in terms of the population's needs and demands for medical care. Health policy has also largely neglected opportunities to constrain total outlays by making greater use of nonphysician personnel in the delivery of health services. Although the United States has expanded its output of nurse practitioners, physician assistants, and other mid-level practitioners, it has never seriously addressed the potentialities of changing the current mix of trained personnel for the delivery of health care services and of relying to a much greater degree on alternative staffing arrangements to provide medical care to different groups, particularly underserved populations (rural and inner city), among whom physicians are disinclined to practice. Rather than aim at replicating the conventional mode of office-based physician practice, efforts to provide ambulatory care to deprived groups might more effectively adopt the models of local clinics and freestanding health centers staffed by organized teams of nurses and allied health care workers responsible for most of the direct service provision under the direction of a minimal generalist physician complement. Such arrangements are likely to offer gains in cost and effectiveness, particularly if the nonphysician personnel are recruited locally and are familiar and identified with the population. A serious reform effort aimed at conserving total dollars without sacrificing quality must direct much greater attention to this dimension of human resources. At the same time it must also reassess and constrain the disproportionate number of specialists and subspecialists that the medical education system has been producing. Physician supply and expanded utilization of mid-level personnel are issues with long-term implications since the worklife of the average professional is about forty years.

A related target of financing reform must be the nation's hospital sector, which accounts for about 40 percent of all health care expenditures. Except for a few states that have pursued aggressive regulatory policies to limit the number of hospital beds and the range of services that each institution is authorized to provide, the hospital sector has been free to chart its future course limited only by its own resources and the funds that it is able to borrow. Excess beds and duplication of costly services offer major opportunities for potential savings in health care expenditures; the approval and authorization of hospital plans for future investments in plant and equipment are even more critical.

Technology, physician supply, and hospital capacity—items that economists designate as "upstream factors of production"—are long-term investments that, once in place, cannot be readily altered, downsized, or eliminated. However, no reform program, even one preoccupied with the near-term reduction of the flow of new resources, can afford to overlook, much less dismiss, these factors.

The final set of considerations in determining the shape, direction, and potential success of a major effort to decelerate the inflow of new dollars relates to the targets it selects and pursues. Should reform address the two principal financing sources: the public dollars made available by federal and state governments and the private funding derived principally from health insurance? Or should the reform also address the out-of-pocket expenditures of households and, if so, how?

It is important to note that even under the centrally controlled National Health Service in Great Britain, approximately 30 percent of all elective surgery is performed outside the governmental system. In most other countries of Western Europe as well, payments originating outside government and insurance—that is, out-of-pocket contributions of households—often comprise 20 to 25 percent of total health care expenditures. Some years ago, the French government enacted legislation prohibiting the purchase of supplemental private insurance, but within a few years the unpopular measure was rescinded. In the United States, a country characterized by variations in income levels and a historic commitment to individual freedom of choice and decision making, it would be difficult to conceive of a reform effort that aimed to impose a cap on all expenditures for health care, including the use of personal funds by individuals who wish to obtain one or another type of approved medical treatment.

Both the European experience and our own suggest that when consumers are forced to rely on out-of-pocket disbursements to pay in whole or in part for a variety of products and services, low-cost as well as luxury items, the demand for these items declines. In the arena of health care, obvious examples are the virtual disappearance of private accommodations in hospitals (the few single rooms that remain are reserved for physician-prescribed situations) and similarly, private duty nursing, the low frequency of cosmetic surgery and the under-utilization of dental care. This eases to some degree the pressure on governmental and insurance payments. In general, health care analysts believe that individuals should continue to be responsible for selected payments, partial or full, for the medical services and products that they need or desire. There is, however, disagreement on the role that out-of-pocket payments should play in determining the demand for health care services. Given the difficulties of designing and implementing an effective mechanism for budgetary constraint in the health care sector, it would appear judicious to allow households to supplement the funds provided by government and insurance.

A second consideration is whether an effort to slow health care expenditures should aim to shift the existing benefit structure from first-dollar coverage or a minor variant (say, a modest deductible) toward greater emphasis on catastrophic coverage, which would place more responsibility for routine costs on the individual rather than on government or insurance. The critical issue is the definition of *routine*. Since a hospital stay costs on average approximately $6,000 to $7,000 and complex diagnostic evaluations often come to as much as half that, only a small proportion of the population would agree to a restructuring of the health payment system that would protect them only against catastrophic outlays. If the immediate goal of the reform effort is to put in place expeditiously a viable program that will moderate health care outlays, the first dollar–catastrophic issue must be tabled. Introducing it into the debate will impede the prospects for reform.

The final issue relates to coverage for the uninsured and the provision of long-term-care benefits. Neither lends itself to a definitive answer. The opinion polls suggest that a growing majority of Americans favor early action to provide insurance coverage for the entire population, although they express considerable ambivalence about assuming any significant additional tax liabilities to pay for it. The elderly and the population approaching retirement are concerned that Medicare does not offer extended nursing home coverage. If either universal coverage or long-term care, or both, were easy to finance and implement, their enactment along with a program aimed at moderating total health care expenditures would elicit broad public support. However, the relative indifference of the public thus far to the remorseless increase in health care expenditures, the erosion in benefits that many will face as part of a major reform effort, and the difficult choices that will have to be made among alternative methods to restrain total outlays suggest that it may be preferable, at least for the time being, to defer the issue of long-term care.

As all successful politicians in a democracy such as the United States recognize, major reform proposals that by definition will affect all groups and citizens can be accomplished only if the majority of the Congress and the voters are convinced that the benefits promised by the new proposals will exceed their cost. The President's skill will be tested as he seeks to persuade both the Congress and the public that his proposals (even with modifications) offer the best prospect for significant gains to most, if not all, Americans.

7

Talking Straight to the American People

Few Americans are informed about the genesis and causes of the health system's malfunctioning, and there is even less comprehension of the preferred ways to address it. In this chapter, we will explicate some of the important factors that underlie the system's growing instability and specify the remedial actions required to restabilize it.

What has happened to necessitate broad-scale intervention in a system that functioned more or less satisfactorily for the past quarter-century without recourse to major public or private interference? True, in the 1980s, the federal government altered its preexistent method of reimbursing hospitals and, later, physicians for treating Medicare patients, but neither action (nor both together) can be defined as a basic intervention in the nation's health care delivery system. Much the same can be said of the diverse actions taken by state governments, including measures to improve their Medicaid programs, the establishment of risk pools to facilitate the purchase of private health insurance by high-risk individuals, and the development of state funding pools to reimburse hospitals that provide disproportionate amounts of charity care. Private-sector initiatives can be similarly characterized as marginal. For-profit medical care delivery systems, both hospitals and ambulatory care facilities, expanded; many employers decided to self-insure; and utilization review and managed-care programs proliferated. Nevertheless, the health care financing and delivery systems that have served the nation since the introduction of Medicare and Medicaid have continued to operate essentially unchanged—with one exception. Between 1965 and 1992, total expenditures (in constant dollars) increased fourfold, from around $200 billion to over $800 billion. Two questions immediately arise: First, what were the sources for this very large inflow of dollars into the health care system? And second, since the dollars have been flowing liberally for over a quarter of a century, why the present concern that the trend may not continue for the foreseeable future?

The health care sector is an economic anomaly: Expenditures for services are governed neither by the market in which the consumer's disposable income determines what he or she can afford to buy nor—as in the case of public goods, such as education and defense—by annual budgetary allocations determined by the respective legislative bodies whose decisions are constrained by the necessity to levy taxes to cover their appropriations. Taxation constitutes less of a constraint on the federal government than on the states since the federal government has the prerogative to generate deficits, as it has done during the past several decades. The fact that six out of seven Americans are insured for some, if not all, of the acute health care services that they need or want is another unique characteristic of health care. It has no counterpart in any other sector of consumer economics in the United States.

Since Medicare was designed as an entitlement program and Medicaid as a quasi-entitlement program, federal and state governments have had little alternative but to meet the steeply rising bills presented to them. Private employers have also exercised all due deliberation in seeking to modify the health care benefits they provide their employees. Like government, most employers have felt committed to paying the health care costs incurred by their employees.

The other side of the coin reflects the mounting claims for payment, submitted primarily by physicians and hospitals, that have operated under few market or other constraints to control the volume of services that they provide even while continuously striving to improve the quality of care that they offer. Looking at the dynamics of the health care market in retrospect, the wonder is not that total health care outlays increased fourfold since the mid-1960s but that, in the absence of governmental and market controls, the increases were not even greater.

Relatively few Americans have any awareness of the implications of continuing health care spending at its present rate with an approximate doubling of the absolute dollar outlay and a 50 percent increase in the share of GDP between now and the decade's end. There has been even less recognition of or debate over the implications of potential governmental action to arrest this explosive trend. Corrective action is indicated in at least four areas to adjust for the disproportionate benefits that now accrue to those at the upper end of the income distribution. Such reforms would not adversely affect individuals in the higher brackets to any serious degree.

The first has to do with the treatment of health benefits by the IRS. Half a century ago, the federal government introduced a tax subsidy to encourage the growth of private health insurance by treating employers' payments for group health benefits as a tax-deductible business expense and similarly exempting the value of health benefits received by employees from personal income tax liability. In the draft of his 1977 market-oriented proposal for health financing reform to Joseph Califano, then Secretary of the Department of Health, Education and Welfare, Stanford University economist Alain Enthoven called attention to the magnitude of this tax subsidy, which he was convinced led consumers to seek more insurance coverage than they needed or would be willing to pay for with their own after-tax dollars. Enthoven recommended capping the tax subsidy, but the proposal was ignored. In the 1980s, the Reagan administration and the chairman of the House Ways and Means Committee, Congressman Dan Rostenkowski of Illinois, revived the issue and sought to limit the subsidy. However, their efforts faltered in the face of the combined opposition of employers and employees. The subsidy, currently estimated to be around $70 billion annually, favors individuals with the highest income tax liability and contributes nothing to the workers at the bottom of the wage scale who pay no income tax. For those at or close to the top of the earnings' scale—executives with a taxable income of $500,000—the subsidy translates (under the new tax bill) into a reduction of about $1,500 in their annual tax liability.

With the passage of Title XVIII of the Social Security Act, all persons eligible for Social Security were statutorily enrolled in Medicare A, which provides coverage for hospitalization. Medicare B, supplementary insurance for physician services, is optional, but the premiums, which were set by a formula requiring 50 percent of program costs to be met by enrollees and 50 percent from general revenues of the federal government, were so attractive that 96 percent of all Medicare beneficiaries enrolled. In the mid-1970s, in response to the encroachment of accelerating inflation on the incomes of the elderly, Congress reduced the contribution of beneficiary premiums from 50 percent to its current level of 25 percent. The cost to the government of this change amounted in 1991 to about $12.5 billion. Although it would be inadvisable for Congress to attempt to reinstate the 50 percent premium contribution for all of the elderly, it could follow the example of the 1983 revision of the Social Security program and seek higher premiums from beneficiaries who pay personal income taxes.

By far the most important potential correction relates to the more affluent elderly, those with personal income tax liability, whose Medicare benefits far exceed their cumulative contributions to the system. The differential is of the order of $7,000 to $35,000, depending on whether the individual's tax payment was based on average or maximum earnings and on gender, with women enjoying greater longevity. Although the health policy community overwhelmingly favored the design of Medicare as an entitlement program, a few public finance authorities were concerned about the potential drain of such a program on the federal treasury and recommended some form of means testing. They saw no reason for the federal government to assume responsibility for the health care costs of the middle class and the wealthy when they reached the age of sixty-five. Since then, however, entitlement has become a rallying cry in the debate over health care in general; a shift in the case of Medicare would be seen as regressive and bitterly resisted. At present, the political, financial, and administrative complexities entailed in such a reform are forbidding. Nevertheless, the issue warrants consideration in the years ahead when the increasingly out-of-control financing of the health care system must be faced.

The fourth target for reform is the use of Medicaid funds to pay for nursing home care, which now accounts for about 25 percent of all Medicaid outlays. Once again, the focus of reform should be the members of the middle class who, if incapacitated, often transfer, legally or illegally, their personal assets to their relatives in order to qualify for Medicaid and thus avoid the high costs of nursing home care. These questionable practices are widespread and result in billions of dollars of incremental government outlays on behalf of persons who could pay all or a large part of the costs of nursing home care, even for a prolonged period.

These potential avenues for reducing government's contribution to the financing of health care will be dismissed by some as politically impossible and by others as not worth the trouble. Such criticisms may be premature and misdirected. Until the task of reining in future health care expenditures is faced and aggressively pursued, these items should not be ruled off the agenda.

There is also little awareness of the dominant role of physicians in determining health care expenditures. Health system analysts have calculated that physicians generate as much as 75 percent of all health care outlays since it is their decisions that determine all the diagnostic and therapeutic interventions that patients obtain.

For example, no one can be admitted to a hospital unless a physician with authority to do so executes the admission form; every procedure that is performed on the patient, from a urine analysis to an electrocardiogram, requires a physician's order; and all elaborate diagnostic and surgical procedures must be ordered and performed by a physician.

Another facet of the interactional dynamics between physicians and health care expenditures is the payment system. Most physicians earn their livelihood by engaging essentially in piecework. This means that the more they do for patients who seek their care, the higher their earnings are. True, a large number of physicians are salaried employees, and many are members of managed-care organizations, where they are paid for treating specified numbers of patients, often or generally for an annual fee, with the prospect of a bonus at the end of the year if the plan produces a surplus. However, fee-for-service is still the prevailing payment mode, which implies that there is a built-in economic incentive for physicians to perform more services rather than fewer.

The predilection for intensive and expensive treatment is, of course, not solely physician determined. Patients who consult physicians seek symptomatic relief—either cure or care. They expect their physician, first, to ascertain what is wrong and, second, to treat them or refer them to a colleague with specialized knowledge and skills to manage their condition.

The recent intrusion of an extraneous factor into the therapeutic relationship has led to a substantial increase in the number of services that physicians provide their patients. In an environment that has ignited an explosion in malpractice suits, many ending in large damage awards, physicians have resorted to what has been termed defensive medicine. They undertake many procedures essentially to provide evidence, in case of subsequent negligence litigation, that they provided the patient the best possible treatment. Liberal recourse to the medical armamentarium translates into billions of dollars of questionable, if not unnecessary, expenditures.

The tort system is frequently identified as the root cause of the costly and dysfunctional environment that characterizes the current practice of medicine, and its reform is seen as a necessary precondition for the elimination of the many "unnecessary interventions" (read "expenditures") that represent a perversion of clinical medicine. When viewed closely, however, the potential of large-scale savings through malpractice reform is problematic, given the fact that patients not infrequently suffer injuries at the hands of physicians and other health personnel and that the injured clearly have need for the opportunity to seek compensation. However imperfect its operation, the right of patients to sue for malpractice is believed by many to contribute to the reduction of medical negligence and to an improved standard of care. Although the malpractice system requires rectification, the solutions to "overtreatment" and "unnecessary treatment" lie beyond the issue of litigation and the elimination of defensive medicine and must be sought in the more comprehensive framework of optimal physician practice.

The physician–health expenditure nexus has still other dimensions. Returning to the assumption that physicians generate some 75 percent of the costs of the health care system, it follows that the number and characteristics of the physicians in active practice are key determinants of the nation's total health care expenditures. In 1960, when the physician-population ratio stood at 140 per 100,000, there was widespread agreement among a large part of the medical leadership, to say nothing of the public at large, that the nation needed more physicians. The delays that many individuals experienced in obtaining an appointment with a doctor, the needs of the biomedical research sector for trained investigators, and the prospective requirement of many more physicians once legislation was passed to ease access to the health care system for the elderly and the poor were persuasive arguments for increasing the supply.

During the succeeding years, the federal government broke free of long-standing precedent and with the use of federal dollars expanded the capacity of American medical schools by about 50 percent, doubled the annual number of graduates, and increased the physician-population ratio to 260 per 100,000. A more moderate rate of increase in the physician supply would be reflected in much reduced expenditures today. Although intensified attention to the physician supply can contribute little to the stabilization of the nation's health care financing during the remainder of this decade and for some time thereafter, any long-term rationalization of the nation's health expenditures must address the issue of the future supply of physicians.

Hospitals command almost 40 percent of all health care expenditures; if nursing homes are included, the figure is close to one-half (46.4 percent). Hence, in assessing where we are and where we should be going, it is essential to focus also on the dynamics of the hospital sector, whose activities consume such a large part of the nation's health resources. From 1965 to 1983, when the federal government moved to a prospective payment system for Medicare, hospitals were in a unique financial position: Their reimbursements were in direct proportion to their expenditures, and third-party payers covered over 90 percent of their total outlays. Hospitals became the envy of every enterprise that had to compete in the marketplace to survive and prosper. Hospitals had other advantages as well. They were local institutions, and most operated in the voluntary sector. In the event of conflict with local or state governments, hospitals had powerful friends on their side: prominent citizens who sat on their boards of trustees. Moreover, as local institutions, they were sheltered to a considerable extent from regional and national competition and were often protected by state legislation that prohibited for-profit chains from entering and operating in their community.

Between the mid-1960s and the mid-1980s, most acute care hospitals, other than those located in declining urban or rural areas, operated free of financial problems. Then the unexpected occurred. In the first half of the 1980s, inpatient admissions declined by an order of 20 percent, as the result of technological advances that significantly shortened the period of hospitalization for many, if not most, treatments and permitted a large number of others to be performed in an outpatient setting. The development of portable and miniaturized medical devices also enabled many patients with chronic disorders to be cared for at home. And the establishment of such legislative programs as professional review organizations, designed to justify patient admissions and lengths of stay for reimbursement under Medicare, was another contributing factor. The much expanded and upgraded hospital system confronted an increasing amount of excess capacity and by the early 1990s, occupancy levels were only a little above 60 percent. Despite this adverse trend, most hospitals continue to report both positive patient care margins and positive total margins. Their ability to remain solvent reflects a variety of entrepreneurial and administrative actions that they initiated. Hospitals entered into new "product lines," such as rehabilitative medicine; they expanded their ambulatory surgical services; and they simultaneously paid greater attention to their billing procedures to take full advantage of the extant diagnostic and procedural coding system. As Medicare ratcheted down on its payments for inpatient care, most hospitals increased their charges to patients with private health insurance. Today hospitals load something on the order of an additional 20–30 percent onto private payers to help balance their books.

Despite the open-ended financing of the U.S. health care system in the post-Medicare era, the federal government made one serious joint effort with the states and subregions within the states to rationalize the hospital structure. Under the Health Planning and Resources Development Act of 1974, certificate-of-need legislation was introduced in each state, requiring approval for prospective capital projects by hospitals for the express purpose of avoiding overexpansion and duplication of expensive services. The planning mechanism was not directly tied to the reimbursement mechanism, however, and in most states, it soon crumbled in the face of opposition from powerful local interest groups. When the federal legislation expired in 1979, it was not renewed. With hospital services continuing to account for the largest source of total medical care expenditures—approximately twice that for physician services—any serious effort to contain national health expenditures in the longer term will have to address both the growing excess capacity of hospitals and the duplication of expensive, underutilized services in the same or adjacent areas. Once the open-ended financing of the health care system is brought under some type of budgetary control and the opportunities for hospitals to cross-subsidize are seriously reduced or eliminated, a sizable number of hospitals will have to downsize, merge, convert, or close.

The high level of sophistication of hospital care in the United States owes much not only to the open-ended financing of the total health care system during the last quarter century and the large numbers of specialists and subspecialists who entered practice but also to the aggressiveness of the medical supply and pharmaceutical companies in developing new technology and new drugs and prevailing on the hospital sector to buy whatever they had to sell. With both patients and physicians eager to gain prompt access to the newest products—once safety was demonstrated—hospitals were under continuous pressure to acquire the latest in order not to fall behind in reputation and prestige.

From time to time, a few of the states and also the federal government resorted to technological assessments to calculate the cost-benefit ratios of specific innovations as a precondition for authorizing them for reimbursement. Nevertheless, the powerful hold of the technological imperative on all sectors of the American public and the open-ended flow of health care funds enabled most hospitals to cover the capital and operating costs associated with their continuing acquisition of new technology.

Two points are frequently made in relation to this technological dynamism. The first is that as long as the United States is committed to improving the effectiveness of its health care delivery system, it must anticipate a steadily increasing rate of medical expenditures, if for no other reason than the increasing costs associated with the purchase and utilization of new technology. The second is that hospitals in the United States far exceed those in any other advanced nation in the amount and level of sophisticated technology they offer. A corollary, in the opinion of many, is that the quality of our hospital care is notably superior. Others dispute this claim; they believe that the nation's medical armamentarium is overstocked with technology of questionable value.

It is worth noting the relative ease with which hospitals were able to acquire new, expensive technology during the decades of open-ended health care financing. A national health care budget, once it is institutionalized (a principal goal of President Clinton), will constrain outlays for costly new equipment. An analogy here points to the unique position of hospitals in this regard. Even in the military's period of greatest prestige and power, the chiefs of the armed services never could obtain as much of the latest technology as they needed or desired. Nor have the most profitable corporations been able to purchase as much of the latest equipment that their various divisions wish. Investments in new technology must always be rationed, and the imposition of a fixed annual budget or some variant mechanism for the health care sector will make this inevitable in the case of hospitals.

Employers and private health insurance have been the backbone of American health care financing since World War II. During this extended period, employers exhibited a distinct (and for business, an inexplicable) indifference to the impact of their commitments to increased employee health care benefits on their profit and loss statements and their balance sheets. For several decades, employers ignored the present and potential implications of annual double-digit increases in their health benefit costs. When they belatedly recognized the problem, the strategies they adopted failed to address effectively the sources of cost inflation, with the result that while their outlays were not braked, access to the health care system was tightened for large segments of the population. Quite early, in the 1950s, employers played a significant role in shifting the private health insurance system from community rating to experience rating, which provided them with a substantially reduced premium cost. In the mid-1970s, they made a second move to cut their health care benefit costs by turning to self-insurance, relying on the commercial insurance industry primarily for administrative services and occasionally for reinsurance.

As their health benefit costs continued to climb, many larger employers decided to control directly the health services provided their employees by means of a variety of techniques that we have examined: utilization control, enrollment (through persuasion or duress) in an HMO or other type of prepaid plan, or contracting directly with managed-care systems, which provide services to employees exclusively through a closed network of physicians and hospitals preselected to control the utilization and the costs of care.

Only one inference can be drawn from the failure of these initiatives to slow the acceleration of employers' health care costs appreciably. As long as the total dollars flowing into the health care system remain largely unconstrained, no employer-initiated cost-control effort can have more than a marginally retarding influence on industry expenditures or on the expenditures of the health care system as a whole. This is the lesson that has emerged from the experience of Kaiser-Permanente, the nation's oldest, largest, and most successful HMO. Although its cost structure has consistently been lower than that of the fee-for-service sector as the result primarily of rigid controls over the admission of its members for hospital care, its expenditure trends over the decades have paralleled those in the fee-for-service sector. Both sectors, prepaid and fee-for-service, have had to respond to the same set of expansionary forces in the health care market: rising earnings of physicians and other health personnel, new technology, malpractice litigation, and defensive medicine.

It is true that individual employers have realized some modest results through the collective bargaining route. In the course of contract renegotiations, many succeeded in obtaining the agreement of their employees to (larger) deductibles and copayments, thereby reducing employers' commitments. It is important to note, however, that these actions represented cost shifting, not cost control.

Paralleling their long disregard of the importance of employee health care benefits for their annual financial performance was the belated recognition by employers of the vast liabilities that they had accrued over the decades for the provision of health benefits to retired workers, currently estimated to run into the hundreds of billions of dollars. Two recent developments have intensified the risks surrounding these obligations. First, many corporations with the largest contingent liabilities have downsized and continue to do so; second, new standard accounting rules require the future liabilities that corporations accrue to be disclosed in their annual financial statements. The initial response of many corporations has been to reduce the health benefits that they are offering preretirement workers currently on their payrolls.

The private health insurance companies have been the indispensable partners of employers in shaping the U.S. health care system. From one perspective, they must be given high marks for having provided for the better part of the postwar decades an effective alternative to a publicly financed health insurance system. However, weaknesses began to appear in private health insurance quite early. In competing with each other and particularly with the nonprofit Blue Cross system, private health insurance companies resorted to experience rating, thereby severely segmenting the insurance pool, with the resulting inability of growing numbers of individuals to obtain coverage at an affordable, or often at any, price, and the deterrence of career mobility through job lock. And in the case of individual policies, excessive sales and administrative costs left only 60 percent of premiums for payout on claims. Meeting rising expenditures through increased premiums, the insurance companies played little, if any, role in seeking to moderate the steadily rising costs of health care providers.

The insurance industry also lobbied successfully throughout these decades against any move by the federal government to assume a direct role in overseeing and regulating their operations. The insurance companies preferred to remain under the supervision of the state commissioners of insurance. The most serious shortcoming of the private health insurance system now is the declining proportion of the employed population that it covers. The growing visibility of the uninsured speaks to the need for urgent reform if the United States is to continue to rely on private health insurance coverage for all or most persons below the age of sixty-five.

What does this straight talk about our health care system add up to? First, there is no control mechanism in place to limit the inflow of dollars into the health care sector. Neither the market nor governmental appropriations sets a limit on the inflow of total funds. Further, it is dangerous to project past trends into the near, not to mention the more distant, future. There is no assurance that the new dollars required to keep the health care system operating as usual will be forthcoming from the American people. Early action to put in place one or another variant of comprehensive budgetary restraint is imperative. The continuation of what is sound and solid in our health care system and the remediation of what is dysfunctional and wasteful are contingent upon an expeditious, effective effort to ensure its future financial stability. Once the financial foundations have been shored up, it will be feasible to address other urgent challenges that deeply concern the American public.

8

Targets for Health Reform

The vast expansion and proliferation of the U.S. health care system during the last quarter century in consequence of the veritable limitless inflow of money established a satisfactory, arguably a superior, level of health care for most Americans. In the process, however, serious flaws emerged, and existing flaws were exacerbated. Improving health care delivery to the nation will require effective actions to address these neglected issues.

This chapter will review selectively major opportunities for health reform that will be necessary and feasible once the financial stabilization of the health care system has been accomplished or is, at least, underway; we will not, however, make reference to their temporal sequencing. Many health policy analysts would object to this differentiation (and prioritization) of the financial crisis and the pervasive structural deficiencies facing the system. A vociferous minority are committed to the proposition that if the United States were willing to confront the extant health financing system head-on and enact a system of national health insurance financed by the federal income tax, this singular fundamental reform would effectively resolve most, if not all, of the other systemic problems, from access to quality.

Such a formulation is conceptually naive. It reflects a misunderstanding of both the American political process and the requisite instruments for system-wide reform. No piece (or pieces) of federal legislation, even as radical as the adoption of a federally financed system of universal coverage that would eliminate the nation's 1,200 private health insurers and relieve employers of their responsibility for providing health care benefits to their workers, could accomplish all the goals that the advocates of national health insurance anticipate. Their primary goal is the assurance that all persons, irrespective of place of residence, would have ready access to physician care. However, most physicians currently reside and practice in areas where they are insulated from the poor, minorities, and immigrants. How would the passage of national health insurance by itself produce significantly improved access for the underserved in the immediate or even the middle term? Effective access might be realized in the long term but that would depend on the implementation of many supplemental reforms.

Additionally, passage of any new federal legislation is contingent on the judgment of members of Congress that a significant proportion—preferably well over half —of the voting population favors the reform under consideration. Once the legislators reach the conclusion that broad-based political support exists, they must find a way to finance the new program, no simple task in the presence of a mammoth budgetary deficit and the statutory commitment to its elimination in the near future. Even if this powerful fiscal constraint were removed or reduced, it would still be necessary to find ways of translating the newly enacted, federally financed health care system into expanded services in the thousands of communities where many individuals currently lack ready access to them. The nub of the challenge is to put in place the mechanisms for translating the new financing into new services. This process would entail the active cooperation and support of numerous intermediaries, many of whom may be indifferent, if not antagonistic, to the new reform.

Moreover, one must not overlook the vast complexities embedded in the operation of our health care system. Approximately 1.5 billion transactions take place every year between patients and physicians (those that occur in the hospital plus the far greater number occurring in ambulatory settings). Unlike other personal services, medical care is a lifelong need of every individual, from conception to death, on average seventy-two and seventy-nine years, for men and women, respectively. Although the need for health care is episodic and frequently unpredictable, it is a direct, personal service that requires a physician to assess and treat the individual patient.

The U.S. health care system operates in some respects under unique conditions and circumstances that help to define the agenda for reform. First, our society has delegated broad authority to the members of the medical profession to diagnose and treat patients who seek their help. No one but a licensed physician has this right.

Second, despite the production of personal health care services primarily in the private sector, by voluntary and for-profit hospitals and private practitioners, the public pays for its health care largely through insurance, private or public. This system is in marked contrast to the ways in which consumers pay for all other goods and services. Further, our society long ago established ad hoc arrangements to provide access to a minimum level of health care services for persons who lack insurance and have no other means of payment.

Unlike any other area of public investment, the federal government has committed itself to large-scale and continuing funding for biomedical research, currently over $13 billion annually, for the purpose of gaining new knowledge that will enable the research community to find the cures—or at least amelioration—for a wide array of chronic and life-threatening diseases. The research is conducted primarily in the nation's research-oriented universities and medical schools (private and public), to which the federal government funnels the major part of its research appropriations through competitive grants and contracts. The findings ultimately are translated into new technologies and pharmaceuticals that are developed for the most part by for-profit firms and are purchased and utilized in the first instance by the private, not-for-profit hospital sector. Given the extreme segmentation of the health care system and its pervasive pluralism, it should be clear that critical as financial stabilization of the health care sector is for its continued effective functioning, it would be naive to assume that financial reform by itself could correct all of the many malfunctioning elements of the system.

We will explore the issues that are critical for a strengthened health care delivery system: universal access, the reform of medical education, alternative modes of physician practice, the reconfiguration of the nation's hospital plant, and quality control. Many other facets of the extant health care system have been singled out for early attention, such as coverage for long-term care, treatment protocols for dying patients, and the coordination of health care and other essential social and educational supports for the needy. Additional topics are strengthened relations among the several levels of government and among the diverse types of entrepreneurship, from for-profit organizations to regulated industries and the not-for-profit sector. In varying degrees, all are engaged in health care delivery. However, for the purpose of exploring the complexities of designing and implementing significant reforms in the current system, the first five areas noted above will suffice.

Universal Access. It is not easy to define what is or should be included under the umbrella of universal access. Presumably universal access means that all persons in the United States, citizens and legal residents alike, would be entitled to obtain the essential medical care that they need, when they need it, in reasonable proximity to where they live. In short, universal access implies removal of the many barriers that now deprive individuals of essential medical care. However, the term *essential* is ambiguous. Once one has specified preventive services, primary care, and acute care hospitalization, there is no consensus. If the reference point is services that a well-insured employee and his or her dependents are entitled to under a liberal package of corporate health benefits, coverage might or might not include dental care; would provide for a modest amount of mental health services (with substantial copayment); might or might not include varying amounts of rehabilitative services; might or might not offer inpatient treatment for alcoholism or drug addiction; and would probably not provide for any, or at best only a modest amount, of nursing home or home care. The term *universal access* is nebulous at the level of its single, essential component—guaranteed coverage.

Suppose one searched for an alternative approach to the specification of universal access. The minimum services that every state Medicaid program must provide are stipulated by federal statute (Title XIX of the Social Security Act): inpatient and outpatient hospital services; prenatal care; physician services; early and periodic screening, diagnosis, and treatment services for children under age twenty-one; skilled nursing facility services for individuals age twenty-one and over; home health care for individuals eligible for skilled nursing services; family planning services and supplies; rural health clinic services; laboratory and X-ray services; nurse-midwife services; and certain federally qualified ambulatory care and community health center services.

Consider at the same time that several states have imposed stringent limitations on the number of days of hospitalization that they will cover for a Medicaid patient. Others have limited the number of physician visits that Medicaid beneficiaries can make in the course of a year. Both the range and the volume of services authorized for reimbursement vary widely by state Medicaid program.

Even in the absence of state action to constrain the use of services by Medicaid enrollees, what is one to make of the situation whereby a pregnant woman is unable to find in her community an obstetrician who will accept her as a new patient, provide prenatal care, and be responsible for her delivery for a variety of reasons: he is too busy; or the Medicaid fees are too low; or the risk of a malpractice suit is too great. There is often an un-bridgeable gap between mandated coverage and the abil-ity of poor people to realize their legal entitlement to effective medical care by a qualified physician.

To complicate matters further, public hospitals pro-vide in their inpatient and outpatient facilities a consid-erable volume of care, most of it to the uninsured population. In New York City, which has operated a mu-nicipal hospital system for the poor since the eighteenth century, annual expenditures are close to $3 billion. Pub-lic hospitals are not alone in providing essential care to large numbers of uninsured persons. The nation's vol-untary hospitals estimated that in 1990 they provided close to $10 billion of uncompensated care. Moreover, all levels of government provide special tax benefits to voluntary hospitals to encourage them to furnish charity care. Arguably, in the absence of universal coverage, a person who receives medical care as a charitable service by a voluntary hospital is not on a par with the vast majority of citizens who can obtain the medical care they seek or need because they have insurance. But in-surance coverage does not always translate into access to care.

Let us take the argument a step further: In consider-ing the challenge of universal access, the issue of quality cannot be discounted, much less disregarded. Millions of poor persons who use the emergency rooms and clinics of neighborhood hospitals as their principal source of care are deprived of any real continuity in the patient-physician relationship, indisputably a serious shortcom-ing in the quality of care that even the most conscientious physician can provide. The excessive amounts of time that patients spend waiting to be seen in the emergency room or clinic of a busy inner-city hospital must also be taken into account when assessing access and quality. And how does one factor in the plight of growing numbers of non–English speaking immigrants who require medical attention but are unable to communicate with the physician(s) and other personnel they encounter in the emergency room or the clinic?

We have already taken note of still another important dimension of universal coverage. The evidence is steadily accumulating that, important as medical care is for the maintenance of a person's health, a no less important determinant is life-style: diet, exercise, the avoidance or use of addictive substances, and other behaviors that can affect health and well-being. We are also beginning to appreciate the potential contribution that ministers, nurses, social workers, teachers, and other professionals can make, in the light of their special training and competences, to improving the health status of selected groups of the population, particularly those with limited income, limited education, and, in the case of immigrants, limited knowledge of their new environment.

These diverse dimensions of universal coverage call attention to the incontrovertible point that, were the nation to make a long-overdue statutory commitment to provide access to essential health care services to all, it would require much additional effort, resources, and cooperation from the leaders of the medical profession and other professional groups before the commitment could become a reality.

The Reform of Medical Education. It is questionable that the objectives of universal coverage could be achieved without addressing needed changes in medical education. A fundamental fact to note is that the nation's 126 allopathic medical schools and its 15 osteopathic schools operate largely under the dictates of their respective faculties, professional accrediting bodies, and the leadership of the medical and surgical specialty societies that dominate graduate medical education and the specialty certification process. Medical school clinical faculties are only peripherally occupied with student instruction; the bulk of their time is spent in patient care as members of a private practice plan under the aegis of the medical school or as staff of its teaching hospital. The fact that income from these activities accounts for about 45 percent of medical school revenues gives the clinical faculty an even more potent voice in medical school policy determination. The dollar contributions of the medical staff currently exceed the combined appropriations of the state and the federal governments for the nation's medical schools.

Policy determination has not always been so heavily vested in the faculty. During the 1960s and the first half of the 1970s, the federal government and many state governments aggressively pursued policies that fundamentally altered the scale and orientation of medical education in the United States. Responding to the offer of federal funding, a considerable number of states established new state schools with the aim of increasing the number of primary care physicians available for practice in underserved rural and inner-city communities. This effort met with only limited success since recent medical school graduates have increasingly opted for specialty rather than generalist practice.

Diverse forces contributed to the predominance of specialists. First and foremost, the leading research-oriented academic health centers that set the style and the pace for medical education have concentrated on the training of specialists and subspecialists. Many prestigious medical schools failed to establish a department of family practice, and even today many distinguished academic health centers do not offer a residency in family practice, despite the availability of special federal funding since 1971.

Once an applicant is admitted to a medical school and once a medical school graduate obtains a residency appointment (usually through the national residency matching program), all decisions that will define this person's later career, such as field of specialization and location and type of practice, are largely under his or her control. The career decision model used by most young physicians aims to find an optimal resolution among a set of competing factors and forces: the individual's preferred field of medicine, the differential earnings potential among the array of specialties, the length of time the individual is willing to invest in graduate medical education, the individual's accrued debts at the time of graduation from medical school and the amount of earnings needed to liquidate them, and the individual's preference as to location and mode of practice. In an environment in which specialists are generally the physicians of choice for the more affluent sectors of the public and are reimbursed more liberally than generalists, to say nothing of the greater prestige that attaches to their work, the cards are stacked in favor of the selection of specialty or subspecialty training and practice in preference to a generalist career.

Any serious attempt to alter this outcome will require, at a minimum, significant changes in the financing of

undergraduate medical education to avoid the accumulation of large educational debts by medical students.
The federal government would have to intervene in the
financing of graduate medical education by using its annual multibillion-dollar flow of Medicare funds to shift
the balance between generalist and specialist residencies. Finally, substantial revisions would have to be made
in the payment schedules for practicing physicians, far
beyond the modest corrections recently adopted by
Medicare. In the absence of such strong-armed societal
interventions, the dialogue favoring an increased supply
of generalists is likely to become ever more intense, but
most young physicians in training will continue to follow
in the footsteps of their predecessors and opt for a specialist career.

Not unrelated to the problem of the underproduction
of generalists is the failure of the medical educational
establishment to have made more than marginal gains
over the past quarter-century in the number and proportion of black and Hispanic physicians whom they admit
and graduate. The continuing shortfall in the supply of
minority physicians exacerbates the difficulty of broadening access to the health care system for underserved
minority populations. Under the stimulus of the Great
Society programs of the 1960s, the federal government,
as well as state governments and the nongovernmental
sector, made funding available to encourage the training
of minority physicians, with the result that the proportion of blacks in the entering medical school class rose
from about 2.5 percent to 7 percent. More recently, however, external funding has been cut back, tuition and
living expenses have risen, and the flow of students from
minority families into medical school has stagnated. The

problem is complicated by the antecedent weaknesses in the educational opportunities available to many minority students at both high school and college levels. Here is another illustration of the nation's unwillingness or inability to back up its professed intentions with dollars and other necessary resources.

Clearly, the medical education enterprise is in need of reforms that will be responsive to the basic facts of American medicine: the interdependence of the medical education system and the practice of medicine, the initial costs of a medical education and the debt repayment obligations that continue to channel physicians into specialty practice, and the special hurdles confronting the United States in increasing the number of black and Hispanic physicians, which is a necessary condition for success in improving access to essential health care for about one-quarter of the U.S. population.

Physician Practice Modes. One of the building blocks of American medicine in the twentieth century was the unswerving commitment of the AMA to the independent practice of medicine by independent physicians on a fee-for-service basis. The age-old code of medical ethics encouraged physicians to treat the poor free of charge or for only part of their usual fee. What the leadership and the membership of the AMA opposed and de facto prohibited as late as World War II was the group practice of medicine, in particular prepaid group practice. Physician members of prepaid medical groups were refused hospital admitting privileges, to say nothing of staff appointments, and were effectively barred from participation in most of the activities of the organized profession. However, with assists from the marketplace, the Federal

Trade Commission, and the courts, the AMA was forced to retreat following World War II, and physicians increasingly were free to exercise their preferences as to modes of practice. Fee-for-service, nevertheless, has remained the dominant practice modality not only in the United States but in most other advanced nations, particularly for physicians who are not hospital-based.

The tensions between the preferred practice modes of physicians and efforts to reform the health care delivery system to achieve more effective cost control are reflected in the recent proliferation and expansion of alternative and hybrid modalities of practice: HMOs and PPOs, medical school faculty practice plans, salaried employment, managed-care networks, and investments by physicians in a variety of health and health-related facilities at which they practice and to which they refer patients. These developments have profound implications for the quality and cost of delivering health care to the American people.

The indolent growth of HMOs before 1980 was in no small measure a consequence of the reluctance of most physicians to join a staff or group model plan that offered a guaranteed salary and the possibility of an end-of-year bonus but required the physician to follow practice guidelines established by the organization to constrain the use of resources and at the same time provide an acceptable level of care to its enrollees. The explosive rise in HMO enrollments during the 1980s was fueled by a new breed of predominantly for-profit organizations, known as independent practice associations (IPAs), which negotiated with physicians in private practice to treat enrollees at a stipulated (that is, discounted) fee. IPA participating physicians practiced in their own offices and were subject to considerably less oversight than the physician staffs of staff- or group-model HMOs, with correspondingly lessened impact on cost control. Many would argue that these second-generation for-profit IPAs do not justify the designation of HMO and are in fact simply discounted fee-for-service arrangements.

In the context of this discussion of physician practice modes, a new option recently offered to HMO enrollees is worth noting: the prerogative to go outside the HMO at the point of service and select a nonaffiliated physician subject to payment of a penalty. The rapid adoption of this option speaks to the resistance of many enrollees in HMOs, PPOs, and other managed-care systems to be restricted in their choice of physicians.

A little-observed development in physician practice has been the vast expansion in the size of medical school clinical faculties, from a total of 16,000 full-time appointments in 1970 to over 80,000 in 1992, and the association of most of their members with private practice plans whose revenues provide supplemental funding for their respective departments and the medical school in addition to covering their own salaries. There is considerable variability in the salary arrangements of the individual medical school practice plans, but in general they seek to devise a basic salary geared to special competence, experience and seniority, adjusted for the volume of the individual physician's billings.

One of the characteristics of these group practice arrangements, formal and informal, is the tendency of the physician whom the patient initially consults to make liberal use of consultations with colleagues and associates. Such ready referrals to consultants can add substantially to the costs of patient care, a practice that the classic staff-model HMO seeks explicitly to discourage.

Since the late 1970s, Alain Enthoven has advocated that employers encourage the enrollment of their workers in prepaid health plans. He argues that the growth of such plans and competition among them, based on premium costs and quality of service, is the only mechanism that will enable the public to have access to essential medical care at a cost that employers and the larger society can sustain. Despite its favorable reception by many health policy analysts, Enthoven's proposal failed to make serious headway until recently, largely because of the disinclination of employers to become more deeply involved than they already were in the financing and delivery of health care services. (It should be noted that Enthoven was a consultant to President Clinton's Task Force on National Health Reform.)

As the result of initiatives undertaken by a number of leading health insurance companies in collaboration with major employers, a variant of the Enthoven proposal has emerged under the designation "managed-care risk networks." In these arrangements, the insurer and the corporate client share the risks involved in setting up a prepayment system that contracts for the provision of services by a network of physicians and hospitals carefully selected for competence and economy.

Now that many, if not most, hospitals are confronted by declining admissions and excess beds, and selected specialists are unable to keep busy through referrals of patients that require their specific competences, insurers may be able to develop and expand managed networks to a point that they become a major provider of efficient services to the American people. However, many physicians continue to be cautious about, if not resistant to, joining corporate networks, and the costs of establishing and managing these systems are not negligible. The ability of such organizations to survive and prosper in a highly competitive, proliferating market remains speculative.

An increasing number of physicians have been accepting salaried positions, full or part time, in order to avoid both the growing difficulties and costs of establishing a private practice and the obstacles encountered in identifying a congenial group in a location of their preference. High malpractice premium costs also contribute to the appeal of salaried employment. The two principal employers of salaried physicians are hospitals and government health care facilities. Although nongovernmental hospitals have generally been able to offer competitive salaries, this is not true for most government medical facilities, which continue to be plagued by problems in the recruitment, turnover, and retention of their physician staffs.

The AMA has reported for 1992 mean physician earnings of $174,400 and median earnings of $148,000. It is not surprising, therefore, that the more liberal members of Congress who are concerned with health policy, in particular Congressman Pete Stark of California, have been investigating the practices of physicians who own or have invested in health care facilities to which they refer patients. The potential for conflict of interest between the patient and the referring physician is evident. However, since such physician investments may fill gaps in the existing medical infrastructure, the AMA has been reluctant to commit itself to their blanket interdiction.

The most recent (1992) effort of the federal government to implement a reformed payment system for physicians who treat Medicare patients, the resource-based relative value scale, a staged process that will not be completed until 1996, is encountering numerous problems. Not a few physicians have simply disregarded the new payment schedule, while others are refusing to accept new Medicare patients, and many are protesting the reimbursement rates that the government has set. These oppositional tactics do not augur well for the success of the effort. Conceivably, adjustments by the Health Care Financing Administration will moderate, if not totally overcome, physician resistance to the new fee and volume controls without compromising the cost-control objectives of the program.

The existing array of physician practice modes is not satisfactory to physicians, patients, or payers for health care. The principal governmental payer, Medicare, is determined to use price and volume controls to moderate its outlays for physician services. Private health insurers have resorted to a variety of devices aimed at cost control but with only marginal success. The elderly have persuaded the Congress to reduce their exposure to balance billing under Medicare as a means of limiting their out-of-pocket expenditures for physician services. The earnings curve for physicians remains favorable, but in the face of patient and payer concerns, the longer-term outlook is decidedly problematic.

While the continuing disjuncture between the financing of health care through fee-for-service payments to physicians and the urgent need of the nation to rein in its health care expenditures remains at the top of the health policy agenda, until President Clinton's health reform proposal is acted on, there are few clues to its resolution.

The experience of the various prepaid and managed-care arrangements in operation is not sufficiently impressive to have produced a groundswell of new enrollees, or of participating physicians should a membership groundswell eventuate. It will take a long period of experimentation to move from what is now in place to the design and implementation of new physician practice modes that will provide an acceptable and financially sustainable level of health care to the public.

The Restructuring and Reduction of the Hospital Plant. With the initial assistance of the federal Hill-Burton program of 1946 and the guarantee of reimbursement for over 90 percent of their expenditures after the passage of Medicare and Medicaid in 1965, the nation's hospitals entered a period of unprecedented expansion and upgrading. During this expansionary era, large hospitals were aided further in their search for capital funding by the willingness of the bond market to sell tax-exempt hospital bonds. Additionally, in the 1970s the new, rapidly expanding for-profit hospital chains were able to obtain substantial equity funding from the stock market on the basis of their impressive cash flows.

The voluntary hospitals, which dominate the industry, have generally avoided price competition, although from time to time they have shaved their customary charges, spurred by an offer of substantial added volume by a major third-party payer. Competition among hospitals has centered primarily on the quality of their physician staffs and the range and sophistication of services available to their attending physicians and the patients whom they admit.

This competition, based primarily on prestige and

quality, explains why so many hospitals in close proximity to one another provide expensive duplicating tertiary services, from open-heart surgery to advanced imaging and radiation therapy. As hospital treatment continues to shift from inpatient to ambulatory settings, it is predicted that before the end of the decade, 75 percent of all operative procedures at community hospitals will be day or outpatient surgery. Accordingly, occupancy rates that are currently below 65 percent will continue to drop, necessitating a substantial reduction and realignment of the nation's hospital plant. It is difficult to identify the processes by which equilibrium between hospital capacity and the demand for hospital services can be achieved. In this connection, it is important to recall that in the early 1980s, most states abandoned certificate-of-need legislation (initiated under the federal-state National Planning and Resources Development Act of 1974), which required hospitals to obtain state approval before making any substantial new investment in plant or equipment.

Not insignificantly, the one in six hospitals of the national total that are currently in financial stress consist primarily of small rural hospitals that have experienced a declining patient load for many years and inner-city facilities with disproportionate numbers of Medicaid and uninsured admissions. The closure of many of these hospitals that are no longer economically viable will exacerbate the difficulties of many poor people in obtaining access to the health care system, for either primary or inpatient care. When hospitals close, practitioners in the area tend to leave, since few physicians wish to practice without a hospital nearby to which they can admit. And as physicians leave and are not replaced, the underserved groups are still further deprived of access to essential care.

A community can respond to these and similar challenges by negotiating the merger of its vulnerable hospital with a neighboring facility or by converting it to a medical assistance facility that will accommodate the remaining practitioners by providing holding beds for patients until they can be transferred to the nearest full-service hospital. However, strong community support, both professional and financial, is required to design and implement such arrangements.

Other barriers to rationalization of the nation's hospital plant and its operations are embedded in the employment and income needs of the local population. In small towns and in low-income areas of the inner cities, the local hospital is likely to be the most important source of employment and income and an important customer of the local merchants. If the hospital is forced to close, the cost in human suffering resulting from the loss of jobs and income may exceed in importance the costs resulting from inefficiencies in the delivery of medical care.

It is more than seventy years since Lord Dawson of Scotland first advanced his plan of hospital regionalization as a means of balancing the needs of local populations for reasonable access to hospital services of different levels of complexity with a cost that could be kept within bounds. With a few exceptions, such as trauma networks, neonatal services for low-birthweight and other seriously-at-risk infants, and burn centers, the United States has paid little attention to areal planning for hospital services aimed at providing optimal levels of care for all residents within a designated geographic area at a sustainable total cost.

Excess bed capacity, expensive and duplicative services, a collision between the economic viability of hospitals with declining admissions and the medical and economic needs of the local population that depends upon the continued operation of its hospital are indicative of the complex public policy decisions that must be resolved. To say that failing hospitals must close is not an adequate response for a society that has acknowledged its responsibility to provide acceptable medical care to its entire population.

In the years ahead, state governments, and probably the federal government too, will be forced to explore alternative ways of rationalizing the nation's hospital plant, at the same time ensuring that no group of citizens will suddenly find itself deprived of access to medical care. This is one more reform, easier to define than to implement, that will be on the nation's agenda in the near future.

Quality Assurance. Early in this century, when medicine was struggling to establish itself as a scientific discipline, a distinguished member of the Harvard faculty noted that an average patient selecting an average physician had a fifty-fifty chance of benefiting from the encounter. A half-century later, a leading New York internist commented that the advances achieved in medicine could be gauged by the reduction in the number of patients who died at the hands of physicians. The current preoccupation with malpractice reform and medical outcomes studies is evidence that issues of quality and competence continue to challenge patients, physicians, payers, and politicians.

Major advances in the quality of medical care have come about largely as a consequence of the standardization of American medical education. The overwhelming majority of medical school graduates, about 80 percent, do not enter medical practice until they have completed at least three years of residency training. Another significant force for quality improvement has been the continuing efforts of the Joint Commission on Accreditation of Healthcare Organizations to upgrade the level of hospital care (recently extended to include nonhospital health care facilities and organizations).

The primary force working for the continuous advancement of professional quality and competence, however, has been the proliferating complex of specialty societies, starting with the American College of Surgery. Their diverse publications, their standard-setting and professional evaluation programs, and their extensive educational programs have led to the steady enhancement of the knowledge and skills of their members.

Nevertheless, there are reasons for concern about various aspects of quality. The medical profession has never been comfortable in disciplining deviant colleagues or recommending the suspension or withdrawal of licensure from impaired physicians. Despite the efforts of hospital management and professional staff in cooperation with external agencies to introduce quality assurance policies and procedures, a recent study of admission and discharge records of hospitals in New York State by a group of investigators from Harvard University found a disturbingly large number of adverse outcomes, many of them caused by negligence, some resulting in permanent disability or death. As for quality surveillance, a recent report by the U.S. Government Accounting Office, *Health Care: Latest State Efforts to Assure Quality of Care Outside Hospitals*, revealed that the shift from inpatient to ambulatory treatment has outstripped state monitoring efforts to license or otherwise regulate most of the sixteen types of freestanding providers that were examined.

Aside from the substantial costs of designing and implementing quality control standards in as diversified a sector as health care, the complementary factors of quality and costs are in constant tension, and on occasion in outright conflict. Consider, for example, the widespread perception that with the passage of Medicare and Medicaid, the nation was well on the way to establishing a single level of care for all Americans. Time revealed that nothing was further from the truth. Aside from major infrastructure differences among regions and localities, wide variations in the availability of care based on income, race, gender, and education persist. No perceptive individual would have difficulty in distinguishing at least three levels of hospital care in any large urban center, to say nothing of substantial variability among clinical services within the same institution. Aware of these differentials and the fact that they are closely linked to the availability of human and financial resources, regulatory authorities are forced to balance enforcement of quality standards with the realities of limited resources, which nonetheless provide a range of services that most communities can ill afford to lose.

Several new departures on the quality front during the past decade have already been noted. The most ambitious, outcome studies, which seek to assess the quality of specific medical procedures in terms of their contribution to the health and well-being of patients, hold promise that improved quality and lower costs may be jointly achievable. However, the potential of outcomes research should not be overstated. These studies are costly to design and to carry out, in both resources and time. There are additional difficulties. In a world of rapidly accumulating new knowledge and new technology, clinical experimentation is a necessary and essential step in their further development and optimization. A premature concern with outcomes assessment could seriously hobble the rate of technological advance that has the potential, with use and refinement, for significant gains in patient care.

A related consideration is that in a desperate effort to moderate their outlays for health care services, both government and private health insurers have imposed a growing number of constraints on the clinical autonomy of physicians in deciding how, when, where, for how long, and at what level of intensity they should treat patients. Adherence to these strictures is required if their bills are to be paid. The earlier societal judgment, prevalent from the mid-1960s to the mid-1980s, that physicians should be free to pursue the treatment of choice for their patients, irrespective of cost, was an idealistic anomaly that could not be maintained indefinitely. However, the current predilection of payers to second-guess physicians has alienated the medical profession more than it has constrained health care costs. The nation needs to devise improved strategies of cost control that will elicit the support, not the antagonism, of responsible members of the medical profession.

With the establishment in 1989 of the Agency for Health Care Policy and Research, Congress became a more active participant in the effort to improve quality. Much of the agency's funding is allocated for clinical outcomes studies aimed at developing practice guidelines for the members of the medical profession. The emphasis on practice guidelines is a potent reminder that improvements in the quality of health care depend ultimately on enhancing the knowledge, experience, and skills of the medical profession in assessing and pursuing alternative courses of treatment. Moreover, the determination of optimal treatment is increasingly perceived as a process that requires the active participation of informed patients, who should be involved, whenever possible, in weighing the risks and benefits of alternative procedures. Like other reform efforts, quality assurance has an important place on the health care agenda. Given the dynamism of clinical medicine, however, it will require many years for sound, practical approaches and solutions to be devised and implemented.

The foregoing review of selected priority targets for health care reform is a reminder of the multiple dimensions of the health care system that require continuing surveillance, research, and corrective action. The widespread belief that it is possible for the federal government to devise a singular program that will provide a comprehensive response to these complex, interrelated issues is naive. Both the government and the nongovernmental sectors must jointly direct their attention to the many facets of the health care system beyond financing that require early reform.

9

Prelude to Reform

It is a deeply held tenet of politics that American democracy typically responds to societal problems by introducing incremental changes in the status quo when it reaches a consensus that change is required. Incisive as that interpretation may be, it does not fit every stage in the evolution of our social and political institutions. Consider the Social Security Act of 1935 or the passage of Medicare and Medicaid in 1965. Clearly there are extraordinary periods in the nation's history when far-reaching, even radical solutions win the approval of the American people and the Congress. However, even radical innovations are preceded by accumulated information and experiences that help sensitize the public and the politicians to the need for major incursions into the status quo to align it more closely with the legitimate desires of the American people.

To understand and evaluate President Clinton's program of health care reform—the subject of the final chapter—it is essential that we review, at least selectively, the principal antecedent developments that have set the stage for the policy debate and resolution that will follow. To lend timeliness and focus, we will begin this prelude to reform with the testimony of the comptroller general of the United States, Charles Bowsher, before the Ways and Means Committee of the House of Representatives in April 1991 on the actions that the Congress might take to reform the nation's health care system, which the committee perceived was evincing increasingly serious malfunctioning. The comptroller general, it should be noted, is the official designated by law to advise the Congress on all matters relating to the financing and administration of federal programs.

In the course of his testimony, Bowsher made three principal recommendations. He advised first that Congress take early action to provide universal coverage to all Americans, a commitment that is inherent in the health care policies of all other advanced nations. Next he urged the Congress to move quickly toward instituting a system of global budgeting, probably the best mechanism for braking the out-of-control rates of federal and national spending for health care. Third, the comptroller general emphasized the need for the Congress to institute a series of administrative reforms aimed at reducing the unnecessary and redundant use of resources connected with health insurance enrollment, as well as billings and payments for physician and hospital services. His decision to present such a radical reform proposal to the Ways and Means Committee suggests that, in his opinion, only prompt action by Congress could keep the U.S. health care system from spinning out of control in the years immediately ahead.

Prior to the comptroller general's testimony in April 1991, Congress had taken two actions that bespoke its growing restiveness with at least selected aspects of the extant system: the adoption of prospective payment reimbursement for hospital care of Medicare beneficiaries (1983) and the introduction of the resource-based relative value scale for physician reimbursement (1989). In the early 1990s both the Republican White House and the Democratic Congress did little more than skirt the growing challenge of health care reform. President Bush stressed the need to alter malpractice litigation, and the Democratic legislators introduced a full panoply of bills, with, however, no agreement among themselves as to the approach of choice.

In 1992 the American College of Physicians, the largest of the specialty organizations, with a membership consisting of more than 10 percent of the nation's physicians, developed a broad-scale program of health reforms that singled out the need for early action on universal coverage and the need simultaneously for effective cost controls. Its endorsement of a system of budgetary controls reflected the members' realization that the large annual increases in health care spending could no longer be absorbed without jeopardizing the effective functioning of the nation's health care system. Not unaware that the introduction of budgetary controls could only have an adverse effect on their future earnings, the membership nevertheless saw no alternative if they were not to risk the collapse of the health care system. The unprecedented departure for a major physician organization that the proposal represented was demonstrated by the vehement attack subsequently launched on it by the AMA.

The American Hospital Association, under new leadership, recommended that community hospitals take the initiative to organize local health care delivery networks that would ensure that all residents would have access to an optimal range of care, from preventive services to hospice care.

The employer community, not surprisingly, was split. Those that provided good health coverage for their employees were deeply concerned about the remorseless increases in their annual premiums, all the more unjustified by the fact that they had to absorb much of the costs of workers in establishments that provide no health benefits. On the other hand, many small businesses warned that a congressional mandate to provide health care coverage would be a major threat to their survival and their employees' jobs.

Finally, increasing criticisms were directed against the health insurance industry for its risk-avoidance practices that prevented many of the most vulnerable in the population from obtaining or renewing their health insurance policies, and against many large medical supply and pharmaceutical companies for their pricing policies directed to reaping disproportionate profits.

So far, the following items have been placed by powerful concerned groups onto the expanding agenda for health care reform:

· The early introduction of universal coverage.

· Implementation of an effective mechanism for controlling the large and steady inflows of additional dollars into the system.

· The potential for significant savings from the steadily increasing administrative costs that consume a large proportion of all costs, particularly of hospitals and insurance.

- Early escape from payer micromanagement of physician decision making, which is seen as an unwarranted intrusion into professional autonomy without any commensurate saving in dollar outlays.

- Reform of the extant system of professional malpractice that has adverse influence on physician location and style of practice and has spawned the expensive and wasteful resort to defensive medicine.

- The potentialities for improving the quality and reducing the costs of providing good care if community hospitals could take the lead in establishing the framework for an integrated system of community care.

- New approaches to moderate the steeply rising costs of employee health care benefits that impair the ability of American industry to compete effectively in the world markets.

- The challenge of eliminating current inequities resulting from the fact that employers that provide health benefits are forced to pay a premium of about 30 percent in their hospital reimbursements to cover costs of uninsured employees.

- The concerns of small business about the potential trade-offs between mandating health care coverage for all employers and risking adverse effects on the number of low-paid jobs.

- The growing clamor about the risk-management tactics of most private insurance companies, which are aimed at avoiding coverage of high-risk patients.

- The widespread perception that constraints need to be placed on the manufacturers of medical supplies and pharmaceuticals on the grounds that their prices and profits are exorbitant.

These eleven items have gained a prominent place on the agenda for health reform but by no means exhaust the list of issues that have begun to attract the attention of the general public or of the professionals and experts who are deeply involved in matters affecting the future directions of the U.S. health care system. Next, we call attention to a group of generic issues inherent in the agenda for reform (no judgments should be inferred about the relative importance of the items on either list):

- All of the serious proposals for significant health reform recognize that a precondition for achieving the objectives of universal access to care and at the same time control costs is the specification of an essential package of benefits that will be available to the entire population. In the absence of such an agreed-to package of benefits, the concept of broadened access would have little substance.

- Closely aligned to the goal of broadened access is the growing realization among the leaders of the medical profession, politicians, and the public that universal access is contingent on the number of generalists who are trained and the incentives that exist for physicians to be available and willing to treat the large numbers of currently underserved rural and urban inhabitants.

- Of growing interest to the leaders of the medical profession and those who pay the bills, specifically employers and government, are the expanded statistical reporting systems and analyses needed to identify diagnostic, therapeutic, and rehabilitative procedures that may not be cost-effective or beneficial. In a health care system that consumes one-seventh of the GDP, a share that is likely to rise in the future, more precise knowledge of what works and what does not is a target of opportunity.

· Gaining attention on the agenda for reform is the issue of redirecting resources from therapeutics to prevention. The proponents are convinced that such a shift would improve the health status of the population and at the same time reduce total outlays since prevention is often less costly than curative medicine.

· Alternatively, support is mounting for broadening the range of mental health care benefits provided by most insurance plans and adding coverage for long-term care. Acknowledging that these actions would add considerably to the annual health care bill, the proponents nevertheless believe that without them, the promise of reform would be unrealized.

· A growing number of informed persons, both medical professionals and the laity, are convinced that significant reforms require not only changes in the financing of health care but parallel changes in the delivery of health care. They see no way of braking the cost spiral and ensuring high-quality care except through a vast expansion in managed-care arrangements, HMOs, and other alternative delivery forms in which both physicians and patients consent to pre-established guidelines aimed at balancing available resources with essential care.

• Fraud and abuse are gaining importance on the agenda
for reform. Estimates as high as $80 billion annually
indicate the need for early and vigorous action. In addition to criminal activities such as billing for services
that are not provided or engaging in conspiracies to
submit fraudulent bills, there are such questionable
practices as self-referrals to facilities in which the
physician is the owner or a partner, dubious coding
practices, mutual referral schemes, and many other
borderline activities that warrant review and control.

Beyond these eighteen substantive issues, we need to
consider at least two additional dimensions of health reform: the major differences among the proposed approaches and the underlying assumptions about politics
and timing that differentiate the principal reform approaches. Our schema will explore the points of difference among the principal reform proposals that, for ready
differentiation, we will designate as competitive market
solutions, the single-payer system, and a public-private
health reform model.

The competitive market model, which in its updated
version goes by the name of *managed competition*, had its
beginnings in the plan that Alain Enthoven submitted in
1977 to Joseph Califano, then secretary of Health, Education and Welfare in President Carter's cabinet. If one
asks why the competitive market solution failed over the
intervening sixteen years to gain broad-based support,
the explanation is easily found: Both employers and employees resisted any effort to cap their tax deductibility,
state governments were skeptical about the fiscal implications of putting in place the necessary fail-safe system
to provide care for the substantial numbers who would

not be covered by private insurance, and the under-development of effective staff or group model HMO structures that were to be the linchpin for the delivery of lower-cost, higher-quality health care. Most important of all was the absence of any leadership group that saw significant gains from aggressively pursuing a competitive market agenda. None of the three principal parties —employers, labor, or government—individually or collectively, were convinced of a return commensurate with the efforts required to go down this path.

The second principal reform proposal, greatly influenced by the Canadian health care system, is known as the single-payer system. As the term suggests, this solution looks to government to assume sole responsibility for financing the health care system; in Canada the fiscal burden is divided between the national government and the provincial governments.

Multiple claims have been made for the superiority of the single-payer system: the relative ease with which government can exercise control over the total amount of money that is made available each year for the delivery of health care to the population; the strategic position of a single payer with control over allocations to ensure that all members of the public have access to approximately the same quantity and quality of services, thereby eliminating many of the inequities embedded in more pluralistic approaches; and the substantial economies in administrative costs and efficiency that ensue from the elimination of competing private health insurance companies. Further advantages of the Canadian system include freedom of provider (physician) choice, fee-for-service physician practice within a regulated fee schedule, control by the provincial governments over the rate of capital outlays for the hospital sector, and reliance on income taxes to raise most of the health care budget, thereby guaranteeing that the more affluent contribute more.

In the face of so many desirable features, what explains the failure of the Canadian model to have had greater impact on the U.S. health reform agenda? The answer covers a wide terrain. For almost half a century, Canada has experimented with and improved its single-payer system; Canada was able and willing to eliminate most forms of private health insurance; and Canadians have greater confidence in expanding the scope of governmental services. Despite the parallels in the respective political and economic systems of Canada and the United States, their populations differ considerably in societal outlook and commitment.

But the real barrier that blocks the United States from going down the single-payer route is the fact that only about $375 billion of the anticipated 1993 total expenditures of $940 billion for health care is covered by government outlays. The remaining $565 billion is paid for by employers and households. Given the strained circumstances of both federal and state budgets, it would be very difficult, if not impossible, for the Congress and state legislatures to assume the financial challenges of opting for a single-payer system and making it operational in real time. A reminder: Canada has been developing and refining its single-payer system for the better part of half a century. And a further reminder: Canada's national and provincial public finance systems have reached a point that both the politicians and the public are beginning to acknowledge the need for assessment and reform. Its public debt is too large, its social benefits too liberal.

This brings us to the third approach, the private-public

health reform model. It starts with the assumption that there are a great many strengths, as well as many weaknesses, in the mixed private-public system of financing and delivering health care to the American people. Its chief strengths are that about two of every three Americans, those with good private or public insurance, have ready access to highly sophisticated medical care practically on demand, with little or no waiting time if hospitalization is required. What is more, the prospective patient has a wide range of choice as to physician or hospital. Its chief weakness is that if two of three Americans have good access to good care, that leaves one of three—the uninsured and the underinsured—without ready access to even essential services. One out of three translates into some 75 million Americans, a sufficiently large number to have commanded the attention of the public and its leaders long before now. There is growing evidence that more and more of the public has come to recognize this severe flaw in the U.S. health care system and believes that it must be addressed and resolved, preferably sooner than later.

Professor Uwe Reinhardt, one of the nation's leading health policy analysts, is an active proponent of universal coverage. He estimates the additional cost to be around $50 billion, admittedly not a small figure but not that big when placed in the context of the nation's total health care spending. A $50 billion price tag for universal coverage would amount to less than a half year's increased expenditures for the system as a whole.

The second major challenge that our ensconced private-public system of health care faces is the early and effective moderation of the rate of new spending. In the absence of such reform, the current system is certain to spin out of control a few years hence, consuming one-fifth of the nation's annual output of goods and services, and all of the three principal payers—employers, government, and households—will be in dire distress, unable or unwilling to continue meeting their health care expenditures.

The third serious shortcoming of the U.S. health care system are the many sources of wasteful expenditures: swollen administrative costs, fraud and chicanery, the needless performance of costly tests and procedures, and the micromanagement by outsiders of physicians' clinical practice, to the disservice of all.

In the face of such serious and growing difficulties, it is difficult to understand why health reform has emerged only recently on the nation's agenda. The most reasonable explanation is that the extant system was performing well for a large proportion of the American people, and although rising health care expenditures have been burdensome to payers, they have had little option but to cope as well as they could in the absence of strong national leadership to precipitate change. In a mixed private-public system, political leadership is always the precondition for effective reform.

The Bush administration gave health reform a wide berth. Confronting growing federal deficits, the President saw little or no opportunity for the federal government to assume a leadership role. Moreover, his principal constituency of large employers, though concerned about their ever increasing outlays for health care benefits, did not encourage the White House to step out front. That was the opportunity that Governor Clinton recognized and seized during the election campaign of 1992. Two basic insights were Clinton's point of departure for formulating a health reform policy. First, there was no feasible way to gain control over the worsening federal budget deficits except by reining in the prospective steep increases in federal outlays for Medicare and Medicaid. Any serious approach to reversing the ominous trend of rising federal deficits required that the rate of federal spending for medical care be moderated. Clinton was the first national leader to explicate the linkage between health care spending and the control of federal deficits. Second, he recognized the growing shortcomings of the nation's private health insurance industry. Through discriminatory enrollment and pricing practices, insurers had deprived a substantial fraction of the public of coverage and had been indifferent to the need to explore possibilities, with governmental assistance, of expanding coverage for the vulnerable population. Accordingly, Clinton identified early the importance of moving as quickly as possible toward a system of universal coverage for the American public.

In an interview as President-elect with the *Wall Street Journal* on December 18, 1992, Clinton stipulated as one of the central goals of his economic program that the nation should be "generally moving toward spending a smaller percentage of our GNP on health care and therefore freeing up much more money for other things." The President-elect continued with the following comment:

> But the people who say that if I want to go to a four year phased-in competitive model [and] that won't save any tax money on the deficit in the first four years but will save huge tax money on the deficit in the next four years, miss the main point which is that if we have a system now which begins to move health care costs down towards inflation and therefore lowers health care as a percentage of GNP in the years ahead, the main bene-

ficiaries by a factor of about two to one will be in the private sector. . . .

. . . I have a big war in my own camp of advisers: Some think we can save about $40 billion over four years even moving toward universal coverage—but that is the minority view. The majority view is that you'd be doing darn well to merely pay for those people who are unemployed and low income that you have to cover by the government, to go to universal coverage.

Queried on his opinion about the imposition of "some kind of a cap on the deductions that companies can take on health care expenses," Mr. Clinton replied: "I think I'm inclined to agree with that. . . . You know there has to be some personal responsibility in this health care system we set up. . . . Once you guarantee a threshold of access there ought to be some limit to utilization."

Seven months into his administration (August 1993), in addressing the annual conference of the National Governors' Association, the President stressed his determination to seek major health system reforms along four axes:

1. *Budget limits.* The President stated unequivocally that the current rate of annual expenditure increases is unsustainable. By the end of the decade, seven years hence, expenditures, if not moderated, will skyrocket from $1 trillion to $2 trillion, from 14 percent to 19 percent of GDP. Such a steep rate of increase will make it impossible, the President emphasized, for the federal government to bring its annual deficit under control; for U.S. employers to improve their competitive position; for state governments to direct essential resources to high-

priority goals such as improving their infrastructure and public schools; and for taxpayers to increase their savings or enjoy any significant increases in their level of consumption. The potential dislocations to the U.S. economy from a continuing, uninterrupted rise in the rate of health care outlays are so severe and ominous that they must be addressed and constraints promptly designed and implemented.

2. *Universal coverage.* The challenge of health reform is that much more complex because of the significant gaps in the extant system of health care coverage for the entire U.S. population, with roughly one-third of Americans lacking health care insurance or adequate coverage to protect them against a catastrophic event. Worse, many with good coverage are locked into their jobs because their insurance lacks portability. Many others with satisfactory coverage recognize that rising premium rates may force employers to shift many of the costs to them or cease funding health insurance altogether. The President called attention to the fact that the growing insecurity of the public about the future of its health insurance together with the free-rider problem created by a minority of employers who do not cover their work force are defects that require early correction.

3. *Cost-effectiveness.* The third critical area relates to the challenges of identifying current expenditures that if better controlled could reduce total outlays without significant adverse effects on the quantity and quality of health care services available to the Amer-

ican people. The President agreed that current administrative costs offer one important target for improvement; malpractice insurance and defensive medicine are further targets; the elimination or reduction of unnecessary procedures is yet another.

4. *Ongoing investments.* The fourth axis of reform centers on the establishment of a comprehensive package of services to be included in the public-private system of universal coverage that will be available to all Americans, as well as ongoing investments in research and new technology that will ensure the American people the benefits of significant advances in the future.

It is probably safe to state that many, if not most, Americans agree with the diagnoses that the President has offered of the dysfunctionality of the U.S. health care system. In the concluding chapter, we will look more closely at the details of the President's proposals for health care reform contained in his historic address to Congress in September 1993; assess the political strategy that has shaped his recommendations; consider whether the reforms, if approved by the Congress, will be able to achieve their objectives; and look past the reforms to the era that lies beyond.

10

What Needs to Happen

The long-awaited presidential message to the Congress on health reform in late September 1993 was a major but by no means the final step in the reform of the U.S. health care system. Systemic reform is a dynamic process that does not terminate with the passage of a singular piece of legislation, in this case universal health insurance, but evolves over many years. The President, and more particularly his staff, have been preoccupied since the inauguration in January 1993 with developing the outlines of his health plan. In consultation with informed individuals, federal officials and others, they attempted to assess the likely reception of the developing goals and mechanisms by the public at large and by the key interest groups whose reactions would largely determine the moves of Congress in shaping a bill with optimal prospects of passage.

Even after the President's program has been submitted, debated, revised, and enacted by the Congress, this will conclude only one stage in the ongoing process of reform. Like the period of prelude to reform, there will be a comparable, if much longer, period of implementation and follow-up. It will be many years before Congress will act on the President's wide-reaching proposal in its entirety. The consequences, anticipated and unanticipated, of the legislation will characteristically lay the groundwork for a subsequent reform era early in the next century, presumably about the year 2011, when the United States will begin to acquire a new demographic profile as the baby boomers start reaching age sixty-five.

A major reform proposal such as President Clinton's health plan is very much a political exercise. It must be appealing to a majority, preferably a large majority, of the voters to permit the members of Congress to support it by putting some distance between themselves and the special interest groups that would prefer the status quo or, at a minimum, some less threatening change. To be successful, a plan for reform must meet other criteria as well, in particular those related to the financing of the new and improved services that it offers. Further, in a two-tier democracy (federal-state) such as ours in which decision making is divided between the private and public sectors, as well as between the federal government and the states, to win support the plan must be tied to a system of implementation that holds promise of fulfilling its principal goals without encountering or creating significant new barriers.

We will begin the review and assessment of the Clinton Health Security Plan by describing briefly the broad outlines of the President's proposals as they relate specifically to the three criteria of political acceptability, financing, and implementation. Clearly what follows is anticipation, not outcome. In politics, timing is everything, and a president who was elected with only 43 percent of the electoral vote is in a distinctly different position from a Franklin Roosevelt, Johnson, or even Reagan who came into office with a much larger percentage of the popular vote that each correctly interpreted as a mandate for significant change.

Only time (the 1994 election) will tell whether Clinton's focus on achieving a radical reform of the nation's health care system, given his weak electoral support, was a judgment that will be vindicated in the political arena. The verdict will depend on his success in convincing the electorate and the Congress that his reform program is responsive to the needs of the vast majority of the American people—needs that no responsible special interest group should oppose.

In his message before both houses of Congress in September 1993, the President emphasized that the core of the administration's health reform plan is the assurance that all Americans would have uninterrupted health insurance coverage, regardless of change or loss of employment, existence of a severe chronic disease or disability, early retirement from work, or self-employment. Once insured, no American would ever again face the loss of coverage. Security of health insurance coverage for every American is the cornerstone of the President's reform plan.

Since just one-sixth of the population is, in fact, uninsured for health care, why did the President define guaranteed lifetime insurance coverage as the core element in his reform plan? The answer is evident. The President and his advisers have become keenly sensitive to the fact that growing numbers of Americans who today have good insurance coverage are uncertain that they will have it tomorrow. The anxiety levels of average Americans about their future health insurance coverage are rising steadily, and the President has decided that the nation must act now to eliminate their insecurity permanently, not simply to allay it for a period of years. That is what most other advanced nations accomplished a long time ago and what the United States can no longer avoid.

If the President and his advisers have misread the anxiety levels of the American public with respect to their future health insurance coverage, the odds are that his ambitious reform program will never get off the ground. Why should it? The vast majority of Americans must be convinced that enactment of the radical reforms that the President proposes will contribute substantially to improving their access to essential health care services. Once convinced, the voters are likely to provide the political clout to ensure that the reforms are enacted—obviously not all of them and not exactly as the President has outlined. Nevertheless, the reform package will gain congressional approval; most members of the House and the Senate will not challenge the President if the electorate stands substantially on his side.

It is difficult to imagine how and why the electorate would not favor the President's plan, which promises every American lifetime security of health insurance coverage, but that does not rule out the possibility of resistance. One reason that the American public might be skeptical of the President's health reform plan would be if it was clearly and unequivocally linked to a substantial increase in taxes or a significant reduction in the health benefits that many or most people now enjoy. President Clinton's Health Security Plan has been designed to be responsive to both of these possible deterrents. The bruising battle the President encountered in getting his 1994 budget approved by Congress left no choice when it came to specifying resources to support his health reform package. It was obvious to the President and to all other perceptive politicians that Americans were strongly opposed to a broad new tax to finance universal health coverage, and therefore the President has had to design his plan without resorting to any broad new tax revenues.

It is not surprising that his preferred option was to mandate that all employers must, beginning in 1997, provide health insurance benefits for their employees, even very small businesses with as few as one to five workers. In selecting an employer mandate as the mechanism for universal coverage, the President recognized that many small employers operating close to the margin might be unable to finance out of current or even prospective revenues 80 percent of the insurance premium cost as stipulated. Accordingly, the President's plan incorporates a number of special provisions and adaptations aimed specifically at small businesses whose employees work at or close to the minimum wage.

One adjustment measure is that small businesses that do not currently provide insurance coverage will be granted a grace period of five years or so before they must comply fully with the new mandate. A governmental subsidy will also be available to assist them in meeting their premium payments. Finally, the amount of the premiums that they must pay in the future will be capped at a percentage of payroll cost.

In opting for an employer mandate, the President indicated the decision of his administration to reinforce the long-standing American approach to health care coverage, that is, to broaden the scope of private health insurance. Further, he has called attention to a serious inequity that exists: employers that provide employee benefits must compete with employers that do not and, in addition, pay a surcharge on their premium costs to cover at least part of the expenditures of employees that lack coverage. To round out the nation's reliance on private insurance coverage, the President has recommended that the tax deductibility for the self-employed be raised from 25 percent to 100 percent.

If permanent health insurance coverage is the heart of the President's health insurance reforms, and a universal employer mandate is the preferred instrument to achieve this goal, the long-term success of the reform plan will depend on slowing the galloping increases in annual outlays for health care services. As the President has remarked on several occasions, failure to slow the rate of future health care expenditures means that the U.S. health care system will self-destruct; the annual increases in health expenditures must be reduced from two to three times the growth of GDP to a figure more or less in tandem with the growth of the economy.

To address this basic challenge, the President has set his sights on several related approaches, each aimed at moderating the rate of new expenditures. The primary efforts involve three principal mechanisms: budgetary guidelines or caps on both private- and public-sector outlays, intensified competitive strategies in which statewide or local health alliances will be able to negotiate more effectively with providers and insurers on behalf of small businesses and consumers, and the recapture of a large amount of current outlays that do not contribute to the output of effective medical services because of fraud, abuse, waste, litigation, and other distortions in the delivery system.

The nation has had relatively little experience with

budgetary guidelines or caps except in periods of war or national emergency, such as the economic stabilization program put into effect by the Nixon administration in 1971. As for the ability of "health alliances" to contribute to the moderation of price increases by exerting greater competitive pressures on health insurance companies and on providers, it must be cautioned that in most areas of the country, such health alliances do not now exist. How long it will take to establish them and make them operational and whether, once they are functioning, they will in fact be able to deliver substantial savings beyond the costs entailed in their operation are unknowns. Their potential to yield the large savings is reasonable but not certain.

What about the third mechanism: the recapture and redeployment of the substantial amount of current health care outlays for services and procedures that produce no useful therapeutic results? The combined sum of these "recapturable" funds is considerable—conceivably in the $150 billion range or more annually. However, the existence of such a high putative sum is quite different from the recapture in real time of any significant proportion of these dollars to permit their redeployment for the early expansion of care to underinsured groups in the population. The opportunities for redirecting some considerable part of this sum should be high on the agendas of both public and private sector payers for health care, but it would be dangerous for either sector to assume that these funds will be available for use in the near term to help balance their current and long-term outlays.

The problematic potential of the plan to decelerate the nation's annual health care outlays takes on added importance by virtue of its intention simultaneously to ensure that the benefits available to the currently well insured are not reduced; to make available to all of the insured a standard benefit package that will approximate those currently provided to workers covered by the Fortune 500 companies; and to add new benefits that will assist the elderly to remain in their homes and that will provide a wide range of preventive services for all.

In order to gain additional support for his reform proposal, the President has agreed that large employers —those with more than 5,000 workers—will be permitted to continue to operate their own health care plans so long as they meet federal standards. He has further agreed that, despite his preference for a uniform employer contribution of about 80 percent of the insurance premium, he will not interfere with present arrangements in which some employers cover 100 percent of the premium cost. And he will allow maximum flexibility to the states in deciding upon their preferred version of the number and types of health alliances, including the option of a single-payer system.

With respect to freedom of choice of providers, the President's plan offers consumers the option of continuing to be treated by their current physician. On the provider side, the Clinton plan is sympathetic to the discontent of many physicians with the increasing intrusion of payers into their professional practice style and interference with their clinical judgments.

The plan has little to say about the largest component of the health care sector, the hospitals, which account for about 40 percent of total health care outlays. This lack of attention to the future of the nation's hospitals whose current occupancy rates are, on average, just above 60 percent suggests that the federal government does not contemplate any direct interference in their operations. Such benign neglect is surely encouraging to hospital trustees and administrators.

In fact, the President's reform proposal has identified conspicuously just one prominent adversary: the health insurance industry. The past and present discriminatory actions of the health insurance industry in the sale and pricing of policies to a large number of employers or workers, the unconscionable overpricing of premiums for high-risk individuals, and the habitual resort to the fine print to refuse payment for many of the costlier bills of the insured are singled out for criticism and correction.

Before we present a trial balance sheet of the President's reform proposal, it is necessary to focus attention on small businesses that will face the greatest challenge if Congress approves the plan with its key reliance on an employer mandate. Many spokespersons of small business contend that its passage will force many firms to close and that many contemplated firms will be stillborn, deterred by the substantial new costs connected with the need to provide health insurance coverage for all of their employees. The claim is that hundreds of thousands, in fact as many as 3 million, jobs are at risk over the next years from small businesses that will close and others that will not be launched.

The President and his advisers do not share these pessimistic forebodings on the ground that their plan has stipulated a reasonable phase-in period, provided employer subsidies, and limited the cost of health care premiums to a fixed percentage of total labor costs. In fact, it is argued that small business has the most to gain from the reform plan, because the proposals offer the only real prospect of containing the future costs of health care for them and their employees. It would be presumptuous to assess in advance of the congressional debate the strength of the opposition that the health insurance industry and the small business sector will be able to mobilize against the President's health reform plan. However, it is unlikely that their influence could be sufficient to overturn it.

What does a trial balance sheet suggest? The President has put forward a major plan for health care reform focused on guaranteeing all Americans, after a specified phase-in period, a permanent health insurance policy that will provide them with lifelong access to a standard package of essential health care services. That is no small commitment, but it is the type of commitment that has been available to the citizens of most other advanced nations for many decades. The ability of nations less wealthy to meet this commitment suggests that the United States should encounter no intractable hurdles in doing the same.

More problematic are the mechanisms that the reform plan relies upon to rein in the rate at which future outlays for health care expenditures will increase. However, several considerations indicate the reasonableness, if not the certainty, that the proposals will succeed in accomplishing their objective. Each of the involved payers—government, employers, and households—is strongly in favor of restraining health care outlays. The President's plan looks to three reasonable mechanisms to achieve expenditure deceleration: government budgetary controls, intensified competition in which employers and consumers organized in health alliances will be able to exert greater pressure on insurers and providers, and more aggressive actions by government and the private sector, individually and collectively, to identify, reduce, and ultimately eliminate the large amount of currently wasteful expenditures.

There is no possible way of knowing whether these approaches will bring the rate of new health care spending within the next four years more in line with the rate of growth of the nation's economy. But the many grounds for skepticism should not overshadow the fact that the President's reform plan is the first to have defined expenditure control as a high-priority national objective, with designated mechanisms aimed at achieving this goal. Two conclusions can be ventured: If the Congress passes the President's plan, the nation will have made the first major attack on accelerating health expenditures; if the mechanisms devised to reduce them prove inadequate, Congress will face the necessity of strengthening them or devising new mechanisms and putting them in place. In either case, a serious start will be underway.

No reform plan that aims at altering the financing and delivery of health care services to the American people that involves one-seventh of the nation's total economy can have identified all of the targets of opportunity and advanced recommendations as how best to achieve them. That is too much to ask or to expect. It may therefore be useful to indicate briefly how the reform program can be enlarged in the years ahead—in fact, must be enlarged if the twin objectives of universal coverage and expenditure controls are to be realized.

There are several important aspects of expenditure control about which the Clinton plan is largely or totally silent. The first relates to what economists designate as upstream investments—outlays for human resources and capital facilities and equipment. The Clinton plan makes only passing reference to the number and types of physicians that the country needs and the scale and scope of its investments in hospital plant, ambulatory facilities, and physician offices.

We have explicated the close connections between the size of the physician supply and the total costs of the health care system. Given the estimate that physicians generate at least 75 percent of all health care expenditures, any serious efforts directed to expenditure control must include plans to limit both the size and the characteristics of the physician supply.

There is another facet of the physician supply problem that needs to be revisited. Despite the large increases in the number and proportion of practicing physicians during the past several decades, large groups of low-income persons in rural areas and in the inner city lack ready access to physicians, who have assiduously avoided establishing a practice in such locations. The promise of universal coverage can be turned into a reality only if the federal and state governments, with assists from teaching hospitals, take a variety of actions to address this challenge. First, it is essential to improve the economic rewards for physicians who are willing to practice, if only for a number of years, in these less attractive locations. Further, concerted efforts must be undertaken to strengthen the medical infrastructure by linking primary care physicians and ambulatory care settings with backup hospitals that will be able and willing to support the physicians who are providing essential care. Unless and until the reform plan moves to ensure that physicians and other health care providers will be readily available to all who need and seek care, universal coverage will remain a promise, not a reality.

The United States has too many hospitals, too many hospital beds, and too many high-priced duplicating services. With the current occupancy level of acute care hospitals just above the 60 percent level (85 percent is considered the optimum), it is clear that long-term cost controls are needed to constrain the (over)expansion of the nation's hospital plant and services.

The third challenge embedded in upstream investments involves policy decisions about the size and direction of annual outlays for R&D, for both basic and applied research and for development. A closely related issue is the investment that must be made to speed the diffusion of significant technological breakthroughs within the health care delivery system. The growing interest and commitment of our society to push back the frontiers of medical knowledge and to apply what is learned to improving health care services to the American people can be gauged by the fact that at the outbreak of World War II, total R&D outlays amounted to $45 million, of which only $3 million was contributed by the U.S. government. The corresponding figures for 1993 are approximately $30 billion overall, with one-third of the total coming from federal coffers. Even allowing for a tenfold rate of inflation over the last half-century, the almost seventyfold increase in real dollar outlays for R&D speaks to the avidity with which Americans are seeking improvements and breakthroughs in the medical services provided to them.

Integral to the challenge of expenditure control is the rate at which technological improvements are introduced into the health care delivery system and are made broadly available to the insured population. Much new technology represents only a minor improvement over existing technology. The implication for expenditure control is the difficult problem of whether the margin of improvement justifies the additional costs. While the United States has been pursuing cost-benefit studies of new medical technology for some years, it has been inclined to authorize reimbursement for almost all new devices that are judged to be safe, with little or no attention to their cost-benefit ratio. A serious effort at national expenditure control will require this bias in favor of the new to be subjected to more careful assessment.

One longer-term dimension of health system reform that the Clinton plan recognized and explored were the potential gains from expanding the population's access to preventive services. The argument was advanced that earlier and more extensive use of preventive services could contribute to both the health status of the population and expenditure control through earlier and more effective treatment. Although scheduled immunizations, frequent Pap smears, prenatal care, timely mammograms, and other preventive modalities hold promise of improving the public's health and simultaneously reducing the nation's total health care bill, it would be a mistake to expect such interventions to make a significant dent in health expenditures. There is nothing on the immediate prevention frontier that points to such a desirable result.

The point has been made but needs to be reemphasized in these concluding paragraphs that what happens in the science laboratories of the advanced nations has the potential of altering profoundly the diagnostic, therapeutic, and rehabilitative modalities that will dominate the delivery of health care to the American people between the opening of the new century and the year 2020, to say nothing of the decades beyond. No one writing in

1993 can list, much less describe in detail, the changes that lie ahead, but they will be large and important. This perception should be a reminder not to become so preoccupied with solving the problems confronting us today that we fail to allow for new approaches to medical care that will emerge in the years ahead.

At the same time that laboratory science is opening up new frontiers, significant advances have been occurring in biotechnology, more specifically in genetic engineering and monoclonal antibodies. These breakthroughs have led the way to a revolution in the targets the pharmaceutical industry now selects for its drug development program. In the brief span of twelve years, from 1980 to 1992, the proportion of biotechnology R&D projects to the total projects of U.S. pharmaceutical companies increased from 2 percent to 33 percent, according to a recent report of the Boston Consulting Group, *The Changing Environment for U.S. Pharmaceuticals*. The same report lists no fewer than sixteen critical disease areas, from hypertension (with 40 million patients) to stroke (with 1 million), for which new drugs are expected to obtain U.S. approval by 1997. The mapping of the human genome that is well underway (with international collaboration) foreshadows an acceleration in the discovery and application of new drugs to a wide range of pathologies.

Even conservative scientists believe that there will be increasing opportunities for early intervention with patients at high risk of serious disease to replace the inception of treatment only after the disease process has become manifest. How long it will take for medicine to shift to significant preventive intervention cannot be predicted, but informed opinion suggests that in a few decades, clinical medicine will be well down the new path.

It would similarly be presumptuous and premature to speculate about the likely benefits in human well-being and the use of scarce resources that will be part and parcel of this transformational process. However, it would be equally naive not to factor into long-term planning the possibility, or even probability, of such a radical shift.

In addition to the increased potential of potent new therapies to address a range of chronic diseases, from heart disease to cancer and benign prostatic hyperplasia, one must also consider the possibility of a substantial shift from surgery to medical treatment. Such a shift does not preclude the emergence of new opportunities for surgical intervention, but if the prospects of genetic medicine were to become clear, especially within a foreshortened time period, the implications for the U.S. hospital and health care system would be substantial. The intent of this discussion is simply to remind readers that medicine and the health care system—more than most other sectors of our economy—are subject to rapid transformations as the result of advances in the laboratory.

The future points to two other potentially important changes in the structure and functioning of our health care system. The first is subsumed in the concept of the importance of life-style for the maintenance of health. There is growing recognition not only among the leaders of the medical profession but among the public at large (consider the reduction in smoking) that the individual's behavior is the principal, though clearly not the sole, determinant of his or her future health and well-being. Genes and trauma, to mention only two, will continue to play a critical role in the ill health and malfunctioning of many people. But illness and disability are no longer seen as acts of God to be treated and, if possible cured, exclusively through physician intervention. The new approach sees the individual as the party with primary responsibility to preserve and enhance his or her health. As this view gains acceptance by both the medical profession and the public, it is certain to have major impacts on the balance among health education, preventive measures, and therapeutics. The last is almost certain to recede in relative, if not absolute, importance.

This brings us to the last of the major transformations that lie ahead, the outlines of which are becoming increasingly visible. The new understanding emphasizes that the environment into which people are born, brought up, and live, as defined in terms of family income, neighborhood associations, educational opportunities, jobs, and other family and societal variables, will largely determine the health status of the population. Sir Douglas Black, the distinguished British physician, has noted that there has been no significant change in the relative health status of the various occupational classes in Great Britain over the half-century that the National Health Service has been doing its best to provide equality of access. The unskilled continue to comprise the lowest category, now as earlier, with much heightened mortality and morbidity.

No one would claim that governmental and societal efforts to establish reasonable equity in access to the health care system for the members of all socioeconomic classes is not a desirable and worthwhile national objective. However, the new emphasis on the importance of environment for the health of individuals and families indicates the need for a broadened perspective of the necessary conditions for everyone to have an equal opportunity for sound health from birth to old age. At a minimum, an advanced society must recognize its obligation to provide all persons with the opportunity to obtain a basic education, to live in acceptable housing, to get a job that pays a living wage, to live in a community protected against crime and violence. Admittedly, it will not be easy even for advanced nations to ensure these opportunities to their entire population. But absent such opportunities, the advanced nations will have to bear much of the onus for shortening the lives and impairing the health of their less fortunate members. Nations with respect for themselves, their past and their future, will do their best to expand such opportunities for all citizens. In our imperfect world, they will fall short of achieving their goal, but having made the effort, they will be encouraged to try again.

The considerations of longer-term developments that are barely visible on the horizon are a potent reminder that the President's two central goals for health reform— universal coverage and expenditure control—are only the beginning of an ongoing process of reform that will confront the United States so long as science rolls back the frontiers of knowledge and so long as the American people have less disposable income than they would like. If the future unfolds in the directions suggested above, we face the following long-term challenges:

- How to alter the training of physicians so that they can better meet the needs of tomorrow's patients.

- How to ensure that even in a new era of expenditure controls, adequate revenues will continue to be invested in both basic and applied research.

- How acute care hospitals will be modified to respond to declines in inpatient care and the rapidly growing numbers and proportion of the elderly in the U.S. population, starting in the year 2011.

- How the U.S. health care system will make room for the enlarged contributions of mid-level health personnel and other professionals, such as ministers, teachers, and social workers, many of whom are capable of playing a much larger role in preventive and community health care.

Important as universal coverage and expenditure controls are to the improved functioning of the U.S. health care system, the foregoing challenges indicate that health reform is a track that has no end. Such reform is integral to the improved functioning of every society, particularly a democratic society that is committed to the principle of equality—at least of opportunity, if not of results.

Reading Notes

For readers who wish to examine in greater depth and detail the major themes addressed in this book, we recommend the following books, which are in the forefront of contemporary health policy research.

Aaron, Henry J. *In Serious and Unstable Condition: Financing American Health Care*. Washington D.C.: Brookings Institution, 1991.

———, and William B. Schwartz. *The Painful Prescription: Rationing Hospital Care*. Washington, D.C.: Brookings Institution, 1984.

Brown, Lawrence D. *Politics and Health Care Organization: HMOs as Federal Policy*. Washington, D.C.: Brookings Institution, 1983.

Davis, Karen, et al. *Health Care Cost Containment*. Baltimore: Johns Hopkins University Press, 1990.

———, and Cathy Schoen. *Health and the War on Poverty: A Ten Year Appraisal*. Washington, D.C.: Brookings Institution, 1978.

Enthoven, Alain C. *Health Plan*. Reading, Mass.: Addison-Wesley, 1980.

205

Fein, Rashi. *Medical Care, Medical Costs.* Cambridge: Harvard University Press, 1987.

Fuchs, Victor R. *The Health Economy.* Cambridge: Harvard University Press, 1986.

Ginzberg, Eli. *The Medical Triangle.* Cambridge: Harvard University Press, 1990.

————, Miriam Ostow, and Anna B. Dutka. *The Economics of Medical Education.* New York: Josiah Macy, Jr., Foundation, 1993.

Rivlin, Alice M., and Joshua Wiener. *Caring for the Disabled Elderly—Who Will Pay?* Washington, D.C.: Brookings Institution, 1988.

Rogers, David, and Eli Ginzberg, eds. *Medical Care and the Health of the Poor.* Boulder, Colo.: Westview Press, 1993.

Russell, Louise. *Is Prevention Better than Cure?* Washington, D.C.: Brookings Institution, 1986.

————. *Medicare's New Hospital Payment System: Is It Working?* Washington, D.C.: Brookings Institution, 1989.

Starr, Paul. *The Social Transformation of American Medicine.* New York: Basic Books, 1982.

Stevens, Rosemary. *In Sickness and in Wealth: American Hospitals in the Twentieth Century.* New York: Basic Books, 1989.

Weiler, Paul C. *Medical Malpractice on Trial.* Cambridge: Harvard University Press, 1991.

The most comprehensive bibliography relating to health policy is found in *Health Services Research: Key to Health Policy,* ed. Eli Ginzberg (Cambridge: Harvard University Press, 1991).

The principal journal dealing with health policy is *Health Affairs,* published quarterly by Project HOPE (Bethesda, Maryland). The *New England Journal of Medicine* and the *Journal of the American Medical Association,* both weeklies, regularly publish important articles on current issues in health policy. The federal government is an important contributor, in both collecting and analyzing key statistical information about the changing contours of the U.S. health care system and in developing projections for future years. The two principal agencies involved in this work are the Health Care Financing Administration, the Department of Health and Human Services (see in particular its quarterly publication, *Health Care Financing Review*), and the Congressional Budget Office.

The other federal agency that is involved in the analysis and assessment of the many changing aspects of the U.S. health care system is the General Accounting Office, which in the course of a year prepares and publishes fifty or more reports in response to requests from members of Congress.

Finally, for the most current developments, the *New York Times* provides substantial, astute coverage of health care issues.

The single best source for ready access to basic health care data is the *Statistical Abstract of the United States*, published annually by the U.S. Department of Commerce, Washington, D.C.

Acknowledgments

This book grew out of a grant to the Eisenhower Center for the Conservation of Human Resources, Columbia University, from the Commonwealth Fund, which I gratefully acknowledge. In accordance with the Commonwealth Fund's practice, I benefited from a close examination of an early draft of the manuscript by a group of invited experts, who made a large number of constructive recommendations.

Long-term support from the Robert Wood Johnson Foundation, the Pew Charitable Trusts, and the Josiah Macy, Jr., Foundation for the Eisenhower Center's health policy studies also underwrote research efforts that are reflected in this work.

My grateful and abiding indebtedness is to my long-term associate, Miriam Ostow, with whom I have been in ongoing dialogue about health policy issues for just short of three decades. Her name on the title page understates her contribution.

Two other long-term members of the Eisenhower Center assisted in the preparation of this book: Dr. Howard Berliner and Anna Dutka.

Grateful acknowledgment is also made for the statistical and editorial assistance provided by Christopher Zurawsky and Barbara Borsch.

Shoshana Vasheetz made two major contributions to the success of this effort: She was able and willing to transcribe multiple versions of my handwritten chapters, and she stayed on top of our computer system to be certain that we were always dealing with the latest draft.

This book benefitted from the extraordinarily skillful, seemingly effortless contributions of Eileen DeWald, managing editor at the Free Press, for which we extend deep thanks.

Index